Public and Community Health

W. S. PARKER

VRD, QHP, MB, MRCS, LRCP, DPH, DIH

Medical Officer of Health
Brighton County Borough

Second edition by

A. M. NELSON

MB, ChB, DPH

Medical Officer of Health and
Principal School Medical Officer
London Borough of Richmond upon Thames

Staples Press London

Granada Publishing Limited
First published in Great Britain 1964 by Staples Press
3 Upper James Street London W1R 4BP
Second edition 1971

ISBN 0 286 62751 5 (Paper)
ISBN 0 286 63024 9 (Boards)
Printed in Great Britain by C. Tinling & Co Ltd
London and Prescot

PUBLIC AND COMMUNITY HEALTH

CONTENTS

INTRODUCTION

THIS small book is designed as an introduction to the vast range of medico-social topics pertaining to the public health. The health of communities is worthy of further study. The following pages are an outline of the work and discipline of preventive medicine. The reader is commended to special textbooks and journals for further reading.

It is the hope of the author that this brief account will emphasize to all students of different disciplines the need to examine the inter-relationship of men and women in health and in sickness within the community in which they live and work, marry, bear children and finally spend their old age. The community requires the advice of a physician experienced in this subject—a community physician.

The author acknowledges with deep humility the opportunity to write this second edition of a textbook created by a respected former chief. I am indebted to my colleagues, Dr Marguerite James and Mr H. J. Pugh, for their help and advice. My thanks to Mrs J. M. Ralls for typing the manuscript.

A. M. NELSON

FOREWORD

THE interrelated problems of health and of disease are not peculiar to the individual; no man is healthy or sick unto himself, for the existence or absence of a state of well-being is dependent, in no small measure, on the circumstances of his total environment, on the places where he lives and works and on the people with whom he lives and works. The maintenance and preservation of his health and, when necessary, his restoration to health are not matters for him alone; without organized *community* effort in these regards, his expectation of life would be curtailed and his fitness to participate in life's activities might often be impaired.

It is with all this in mind that this textbook has been prepared both for the undergraduate and the post-graduate student of medicine alike, in order that they be given a wide vision and understanding of what medicine means and of how fully it may contribute to the health and happiness of mankind, and of its place outside the four walls of the hospital or consulting room.

A familiarity with the rise, growth and development of the public health, the industrial health and the social services, not only in the national but also in the international field, is an *essential* part of the full education of the medical student at university level. He should know and appreciate all that is done by local authorities and other bodies in the furtherance of the nation's health and of the help and assistance which is being made available to the physically, mentally and socially handicapped as well as to the aged in our midst. Such an extension of his professional education, which must not be wholly limited to bedside instruction, will not only increase his stature as a true physician, that is as a student of man in his relation to nature, but will also open his mind to the fact that the public and industrial health services, together with the allied social services, are complementary to and not in competition with clinical medical practice.

Public and Community Health is a valuable contribution to medical education. Its use in all schools of medicine would help

xi

to remove the impression that at times the nurturing of the medical student in the aims and purposes of social and preventive medicine is undoubtedly lacking.

NEIL R. BEATTIE
Dean
Royal Institute of Public Health and Hygiene

PREFACE TO THE FIRST EDITION

THIS small book is planned as an introduction to the vast range of medico-social topics which make up Public Health as we know it in this country. As community health must involve occupational health a short chapter has been included on this subject.

The following pages are an outline of the work and discipline of preventive medicine including those aspects which directly concern the National Health Service. The reader is commended to the various special textbooks and journals for further reading.

It is the hope of the author that this brief account will emphasize to the medical student the need for study of the interrelationship of men and women in health and in ill health within the community in which they live and work, marry, bear children and finally spend their old age. It may induce in the student the idea that disease and misery ought not to exist and that, with forethought, much of it can and should be prevented.

In presenting this book to the reader I would wish to acknowledge the help and advice which I have received from Dr A. M. Nelson, my former Deputy, his successor Dr W. H. Allen, and from the senior members of the Brighton Health Department, in particular Mr H. G. Gibson, Deputy Chief Public Health Inspector, who read the proofs of the environmental section. My wife, Dr Margaret Parker, read the book and made many helpful suggestions. My secretary, Mrs G. R. Bennett, coped with the manuscript.

I am particularly indebted to Dr H. D. Chalke, o.b.e., Medical Officer of Health of Camberwell, for his kind permission to quote extensively from the recent book on Radiation and Health of which he is the co-author. In conclusion, I wish to thank Dr Neil Beattie for so kindly agreeing to write the Foreword to my book.

W. S. PARKER

PREFACE TO THE SECOND EDITION

THE health of communities is worthy of further study. All students of different disciplines need to examine the interrelationship of men and women in health and in sickness within the community in which they live and work, marry, bear children, and finally spend their old age.

For over a century the exponents of public health have been striving with much success to achieve certain basic requirements for a community. These are a pure water supply, reliable sewage and refuse disposal systems, clean food, adequate sound shelter and clean air. The horizons are widening to take in the notion of conservation of the environment. These aims are now current topics, even at international level. The study of the spread and control of infectious disease involves a partnership between the sciences of epidemiology and bacteriology.

Society understands and agrees measures to control contagion. Social medicine studies the epidemiology of the non-infectious disease, the causation of sickness and the delivery of health care services.

Hospitals investigate and treat patients on either an in- or outpatient basis and thus serve the community at large. The patient in a hospital bed, having been removed from his own home, is cared for, nursed, and treated by a professional staff to a very high order. The hospital service, in many parts of the world, holds a high proportion of resources both in finance and personnel. The community outside the hospital walls also cares for, nurses and treats sick people. Personal physicians and community nurses undertake these tasks in the patient's own home in collaboration with relatives, neighbours and friends. It is being postulated that there is a newer discipline—that of community medicine, the parameters of which are evolving. A medical practitioner with appropriate experience and training who advises the community could be termed a community physician—the physician to the community. The objects of his concern are social obstetrics and paediatrics and the presymptomatic diagnosis of disease, with particular emphasis on the concept of vulnerability to physical, mental and social risks. In addition, those diseases with a social causation and therapy must be considered.

Of acute moment is the interface between health and social services. The improvement of community health in the environment is studied.

A. M. NELSON

Part One   Community Health

I

Community Health

WHEREVER man has been able to organize his activities the resultant functioning structure can be considered as a society, however primitive it may be. Many individuals will live, work and play in harmony within such a society. However, a minority will be in disharmony with their society. This disharmony can lead to social degeneration, which is a fertile nidus for disease. Conversely disease may be the cause. Medicine is deeply concerned, whatever the cause.

The techniques of medicine have now achieved a high degree of sophistication and expertise with resultant benefits to mankind. The practice of medicine is a highly respected paradox in that a skilful scientific discipline is pursued as an art moulded by humanity, humility and compassion. Medicine is involved in the causation, identification and treatment of disease and disability. The latter in a limited concept is considered by some to involve either surgical intervention or the prescribing of 'pills and potions'.

Medicine concerned with the disharmony in society is a social science in its own right, although the ensuing therapy may have a purely social basis. This therapy may be administered not by medical men alone, but also by others, e.g. engineers, architects, lawyers, educationists and social workers. Medicine is involved in the writing of the social prescription, but medical men do not necessarily dispense this prescription. We see therefore that medicine, in partnership with other disciplines, aims to eradicate social disharmonies.

Evolving society calls for the provision of abundant food supplies, pure water, adequate shelter and satisfactory refuse and sewage disposal. This state of affairs is not always achieved. If these environmental requirements are non-existent or function in a limited way, then disease and pestilence will flourish. Medical men, with others, have combated these pestilences by following the sanitary sciences. The structure of society determined that a strict sanitary policy approach should be adopted to control infectious disease, eradicate bad housing and overcrowding, provide

3

pure water, and safe refuse disposal. Thus the discipline of the public health services was born. The science of bacteriology was the foundation of the study of infectious disease transmitted from one individual to another in a community, known as epidemiology—the study of epidemics.

As environmental factors in disease causation improve, medicine seeks out the incidence of non-infective disease and studies the organization of medical care. This science is the academic discipline of social medicine.

For many centuries the sick received tender, loving care in hospices. From the concentration of this compassion and nursing in such establishments has evolved the modern hospital service.

Two streams of medicine appear to have been created. On the one hand, there is the medicine of the hospital world, concerning itself with sick people in beds within hospital walls, where professionals treat those individuals who have been removed from the community outside the hospital walls. Such medicine tends to have a technological approach. On the other hand, there are many sick people who remain in the 'world of the well'. They are often old, and have an impaired or disturbed mental state, or are disabled physically. Thus a style of medicine exists which has a sociological approach—seeking out and supporting sick individuals within the community. A newer and controversial medicine, whose parameters are not yet clearly defined, is now forming; this discipline could be described as community medicine, i.e. the practice of medicine within the community, where the therapy may well be social.

Whenever a set of social circumstances are disturbing and need resolving, men and women of good will join together to examine the unsatisfactory state of affairs. Medical practitioners may be so involved. A voluntary group forms, with one of its aims to alter and guide public opinion. In any debate there will be a basic medical recommendation in either a positive or negative form. As public opinion crystallizes, a social policy evolves, on which political action can be determined.

This thesis and cycle of basic medical recommendation, the evolution of social policy and resultant action, in some instances political, can be applied to the individual, family, community and even the nation.

Social policies which disregard adequate medical recommendation are doomed to either total or partial failure. Medical men must appreciate the high public regard of their advice, but also be wary, for they can only achieve the ultimate elimination of social disharmony by partnership with others, be they sociologists or politicians.

The traditional pillars on which public health practice is founded are concerned with the procurement of a hazard-free environment for the community. These aims are as important as ever today, be they in an advanced community or a developing society.

An adequate and safe water supply is the most important community health requirement. Water is used for drinking, for community services, for agriculture and for industry. In any developing community an irreversible and increasing demand can be predicted. The arrangements for supply must be planned with full anticipation of what will be required in future years.

After water, food is the next essential for survival. An adequate diet in itself is one of the most important contributions to public health. With advances in agriculture and fishing, surplus food is stored and can be traded. Trade means communication; communication means change. Agriculture and industry and communication alter public health problems.

Personal protection by clothing and family protection against the elements in a dwelling are the most immediate needs when hunger and thirst are satisfied. Both climate and cultural habits are involved. The gregarious habits of man, the adoption of specialized occupations and the growth of trade routes, all contribute to the creation, siting, design and conduct of the homes and other buildings in the community. Into this is woven a complex pattern of psychological needs, achievements, stresses and frustrations, all of which emphasize the significance of the mental health aspect of community life.

Public health problems of sewage and refuse disposal arise whenever a group of people live together. Traditional usage cannot necessarily be relied upon to supply a satisfactory answer. It is more than probable that any existing community refuse disposal plan could be improved on grounds of health.

Some form of education goes on in all communities. It ranges from teaching by tribal elders or by the local priest to a full modern system of education. One phenomenon must be mentioned. The rate of progress is not the same throughout the world. Such is the rate of apparent acceleration in some underdeveloped countries at the present time that ideas have outpaced literacy. Failing the stabilizing influence of the individual's being able to reflect and to re-read about the topic of interest, some alternative basis for the education and training of the general population must be found. This need for a new fundamental medium of communication and instruction is a problem of paramount importance to all concerned.

In primitive communities few matters are more hedged about by tradition and superstition than is medicine, universally involved in the mysteries of birth and death. The most tactful and thorough health education is necessary to introduce modern preventive and clinical practice. Though the prevention of disease will achieve greater successes in the long run, it is essential that some curative services be provided at the outset and expanded to meet local needs. By securing confidence in modern healing practice the initial status of preventive medicine is raised and a climate of acceptance is created for future epidemiological and sanitary measures.

Thus a preventive ideal must be maintained and enhanced at all times.

Study of Population

The study of population is known as demography. A population is not a static entity but is in a fluid state both as to quality and quantity. An essential base line is the 'counting of heads' or in official parlance, the taking of a census at periodic intervals. The total number of individuals in a given population is thus determined. As to quantity, a population is increased by natality and immigration. A population is decreased by mortality and emigration.

Thus a population can be estimated for inter-census years by applying the indices of natality, mortality and migration. The difference between the sum of the births and immigrants and the sum of deaths and emigrants will give the actual increase or decrease in a given population.

As to quality, the genetical endowment and experience of those who leave a population by death or emigration are never identically replaced by the gifts of those who enter that population by birth and immigration. Thus the structure of a population can be based on its age and sex components. Entry to this design is by birth and departure is by death. There follow three main groupings:

    (1) Immatures   Birth–15 years
    (2) Matures   16 years–64 years
    (3) Elderly   Over 65 years

An individual passes from the immature to mature group. Entry to the elderly grouping can only be from the matures. The size of each group in relation to the others is a vital factor in a society. The mature group supports the other two.

The mean age of a population can be determined by taking the sum of the ages of the individuals divided by the total number of individuals. A population with a low mean age has a large immature group. A population with a high mean age has a large elderly component. When over a period of years the mean age rises, then an ageing population exists.

Society, to plan services for health, education and housing at either local, regional or national level, must look critically at the population concerned with these groupings of immatures, matures, and elderly in mind.

As the composition of one population is always different in quality and quantity from that of another, it follows that a comparison of the number of births and/or deaths between the populations is not a true reflection of the circumstances. Therefore a rate is determined in relation to a given common factor of, say, one thousand population. Therefore the following formulae are important:

$$\text{Crude Birth Rate} = \frac{\text{Number of live births registered in the year} \times 1000}{\text{Estimated mid-year population}}$$

40–50 per thousand in developing areas. 15–20 per thousand in advanced communities.

$$\text{Crude Death Rate} = \frac{\text{Number of deaths registered during the year} \times 1000}{\text{Estimated mid-year population}}$$

40 per 1000 in developing areas. 10 to 20 per 1000 in highly civilized communities.

The evolution of a population follows a given demographic cycle and every population is fluctuating, however slowly, from phase to phase in that cycle.

Phase 1. The most elementary community has very limited safeguards against famine and pestilence and does not take advantage of periods of plenty. A high birth rate and a high death rate operate at the same time. The population is therefore static.

Phase 2. A society organizes food production and storage. Sanitary disciplines are established. The forces of good are capitalized, and the forces of adversity contained. The birth rate remains high. The death rate decreases. A natural increase ensues.

Phase 3. The social standards rise. Medical care exerts its influence. The birth rate falls a little, but the death rate falls faster. The natural increase in population is marked. The mean average age of the population is low.

Phase 4. The society is much more complex. Health services are sophisticated. The birth rate is lower. When every woman in the reproductive age period is reproduced, the reproductive index is unity. In this phase the index fluctuates marginally around unity. The death rate also is low.

Phase 5. The death rate is higher than a low birth rate. An ageing population is reflected in a rising mean average age. The ultimate situation is the extinction of the population. These circumstances are described as the depopulation of an area.

The well-being of a people is reflected by these natural forces, which are the most sensitive indices of social and political activities.

REFERENCES

Crew, F. A. E. (1948) *Measurements of the Public Health* (Oliver and Boyd, Edinburgh and London).
Smith, Alwyn (1968) *The Science of Social Medicine* (Staples Press, London).
Vickers, G. (1967) *Lancet*, I, 944.

2

Social Obstetrics

SOCIETY has determined that the creation and stability of a family biologically must be maintained within the religious, moral, and legal ties of marriage. The vast majority of communities follow the code of monogamy, although polygamy is practised, within certain safeguards, in different parts of the world. If the latter is not the established custom then dissolution of the monogamous marriage by divorce is accepted in many societies, though not always with religious approval. The successful outcome of the biological union in marriage is the progress of conception, pregnancy and the ultimate birth of a live infant. However, the sanctity and purpose of marriage is being questioned in certain cultures, and more elementary associations and stable relationships are being attempted. So much so that both inside and outside marriage, conception and pregnancy have been described in certain individuals as a means of escape from reality.

Promiscuity can be defined as a sexual relationship by one individual with more than one partner, both inside and outside marriage. In any study of promiscuity there are no known direct measurements, only indirect indices, which can only indicate trends. Extra-marital sexual intercourse can result in conception and subsequent birth of an infant outside wedlock, which can be expressed as a percentage of the legitimate births. An imperfect index of pre-marital intercourse is the number of births occurring within nine months of marriage. A number of factors can invalidate these indirect indices.

1. The knowledge, availability and expertise in contraceptive practices.
2. The availability, attitudes and acceptability of the techniques in termination of pregnancy.
3. The influence of alcohol and drugs.
4. The religious and cultural *mores* of the community concerned in relation to 'shot-gun marriage'.
5. Fertility. Some individuals are more fertile with one partner than with another.

9

6. False declarations can be made on a marriage certificate.
7. Married women have the opportunity of conceiving with a male consort and registering the subsequent birth in the name of the husband. Thus to society the child is born within wedlock, though biologically conceived outside.

Venereal disease is the social disease *par excellence*. The social aspect takes two main lines. Firstly, there is the debasement of sexual union as a supreme experience, with consequent lowering of the community value of the marriage-bond and all that it implies, either as sought by the single or maintained by the married. Secondly, there are the direct results of infection usually by syphilis or gonorrhoea.

Quite apart from the personal consequences, the immediate hazard is the further spread of infection by a promiscuous patient in an infective condition. The results in the patient are well known: in gonorrhoea the discomfort and difficulty of being an ambulant patient, the hazard to the eyesight and the further disabilities of arthritis and of urethral stricture in the male. In the female the symptoms are slight. She may not know she has been infected but the consequences include sterility, which has a social bearing on the future of the community, and the risk of infection of the infant at the moment of birth, with resultant blindness from *ophthalmia neonatorum*.

Syphilis can be acquired or inherited. The disease frequently goes unrecognized in women as the primary lesion is not seen. The social consequences of neglect or ineffective treatment are tragic. The neurological consequences of syphilis are disability and mental derangement. The infant which inherits syphilis acquires disabilities and deformities to brain, bone, soft tissues and physique which can never be wholly remedied. As both diseases are preventable they are in theory completely avoidable. The social effects fall on the individual or on to the community, which must maintain the sufferer either directly or implicitly by having to accept his inefficient presence in its midst in the knowledge that with proper care or continence the infection need not have occurred.

While the majority of pregnancies occurring within marriage are planned as mutually initiated biological events, a substantial minority proportion are unplanned. Measures which are contraconception, and so preventing conception, are given the abbreviated term contraception.

Knowledge of these measures is very variable and is dependent on moral, religious, and practical customs and experience. This knowledge and its implementation is the potential preventive measure for certain social ills. These are the unplanned results of promiscuity; the economic burden amounting to poverty brought about by many children born in rapid succession; maternal morbidity; marital disharmony and strained family dynamics. The balance in the world between population growth and food supplies can be precarious. Slowing down and reversing the former in an attempt to correct imbalance can be achieved in population control programmes with the active teaching of contraceptive techniques as the prime preventive step. At the family level, the resources of the biological unit may be able to cope adequately with one or two children. If, however, a third or subsequent pregnancy follows at too short an interval, then poverty can ensue. Contraceptive measures could well avoid these circumstances. The fear of another pregnancy can strain a marriage to its breaking point. The husband may be tempted to seek his sexual needs and satisfactions with another consort, on either a transient or permanent basis.

Relationships in the young can be jeopardized rather than enhanced by an unplanned pregnancy. Several alternative consequences can ensue:

1. Termination of the pregnancy, sometimes under unsuitable circumstances with disastrous physical and emotional consequences.
2. 'Shot-gun' marriage—the majority fraught with emotional family tensions, which may, however, resolve in time.
3. An unsupported mother, at social risk, earning her own living to support a bastard.

Knowledge of contraceptive techniques could well have averted these social catastrophes. However, this specific knowledge is only part of an awareness of human relationships, including personal responsibility. Any educative programme must take this broad view. The words used in such communication may on the one hand be sophisticated medical terms, or on the other hand be crude, earthy, obscene slang.

The methods of contraception range from complete abstinence to complex hormonal control. The emphasis and main responsibility tends to rest solely with the female. Mechanical and chemical barriers are used singly or together. The hormonal method by mouth for women, 'The Pill', has simplicity, but certain minimal complications have not yet been resolved. The social effect of this method has yet to be measured, but its potential for good is immense. Ligation of the *vas deferens* is a permanent method for the male, and within certain criteria has its place.

A pregnancy may terminate itself by foetal death. The resultant inevitable miscarriage may be spontaneous, complete or partial. A partial inevitable miscarriage needs to be completed by surgical intervention. The mental and physical health of the mother can be put at risk by the advent and presence of a pregnancy. The foetus may possess certain hereditary abnormalities or develop congenital defects, which would have severe handicapping results. Within these broad indications termination of the pregnancy is a therapeutic measure. Abortion carries the risk of death and ill health, due to haemorrhage and infection, particularly if it is carried out by unqualified operators under primitive conditions, and even if practised by highly skilled and qualified gynaecological surgeons in well-equipped hospital theatres.

Some argue that there are pure social grounds for termination of pregnancy. This reasoning is unacceptable to many medical practitioners. In many of the alleged social instances a sound medical reason can be found, and the resultant therapeutic termination is clinically valid. If no medical reason is forthcoming, then the pregnancy should continue.

By whatever means the termination is achieved, the emotional trauma due to loss of a potential live infant is severe. The woman on the surface may deny such emotional involvement and present a courageous front to relatives and friends. This emotional trauma calls for sympathy, understanding and support by her professional attendants and members of the society and culture in which she lives. Whatever may be the grounds for the termination, whatever the age of the patient, whatever the moral culture of the community, contraceptive advice in both general and particular terms should be offered, lest a subsequent unplanned pregnancy should follow at a short interval. The medical attendant is failing in his professional obligation to his patient if this after-care is not given careful consideration.

The pregnant woman is entitled to scrupulous antenatal care, for both her own future well-being and that of her infant. Periodic regular examination and assessment by both professional medical and midwifery personnel is axiomatic for this care so that deviations from good health can be detected and corrected. Advice on diet, rest and relaxation can be given and clinical features of impending and underlying pathology treated. Such antenatal care can be organized either by the physician of first contact or by the midwife at a surgery or clinic. The maternity hospital where the subsequent delivery will take place always provides antenatal care on an out- and in-patient basis. An integral part of this care is the preparation for labour and early infant management. The professional attendants must discuss, and advise the mother on, the place of delivery, equipment, and procedures involved. The trend in both civilized and primitive communities is from domiciliary confinements to delivery in hospital. The reasoning being that the mother thus has a hazard-free delivery. After a trouble-free labour, a gradually active puerperium is advocated before the mother returns to her domestic commitments. Legislation exists in certain communities to restrain women from continuing to work during the later stages of pregnancy and from returning to gainful occupations too early. On social and psychological grounds the advantages of a home confinement are attractive in civilized communities for the second and third pregnancy. The anxiety to the mother of a break in her relationship with the older children is minimized. The relationship between the siblings is strengthened at a very early stage.

Balancing the hazard-free and safe hospital delivery against these arguments for a stable emotional state in the family has led to schemes of planned early hospital discharges. The mother, cared for by either her personal professional attendants or by hospital staff, is delivered in a maternity unit, remains for a short period of say, twelve, twenty-four, or forty-eight hours, and returns home. These schemes are dependent on flexible professional attitudes, good will, sound transport systems, adequate domestic help from relatives and others, and home conditions of good standard.

Complementary to antenatal care is parentcraft teaching, especially mothercraft. Fathers must not be excluded from this basic facet of health education.

Socio-medical services must be so structured that the unsupported mother, be she unmarried, widowed, or separated from her husband, receives her antenatal care, since she is at medical and social risk. If she has left her home, as with the unmarried, special hostel or sheltered flatlet accommodation is necessary during the last trimester of pregnancy. She leaves this home temporarily, to be delivered in hospital and subsequently returns to its shelter.

It is a truism that sound obstetric practice is preventive gynae-cology. Therefore it follows that all puerperal women should receive detailed postnatal follow-up for six to twelve weeks after delivery. Any pathological clinical lesion so discerned can be treated. Marital and contraceptive counselling is an essential feature of the postnatal check.

An index of the quality of maternity care services, as well as the living standards of the community, is the number of maternal deaths. The maternal mortality rate can be defined in two parts:

1. Those deaths due to truly puerperal causes—puerperal causes.
2. Those deaths due to other pathological causes in a woman who was pregnant at the time—associated causes.

The puerperal (maternal) mortality rate is the number of deaths in the year ascribed to pregnancy and childbirth per 1,000 confine-ments. The associated (maternal) mortality rate is the number of deaths of women in the year (per 1,000 confinements) ascribed to causes other than puerperal, but operating in pregnancy and being reinforced by the hazards of pregnancy and childbirth.

In England and Wales each maternal death is subjected to a detailed confidential inquiry by the professional attendants con-cerned. Each questionnaire is examined by a highly experienced obstetrician. Every three years the observations, results, and recommendations on the findings are published. These reports are essential reading for all students of social obstetrics.

REFERENCES

Ministry of Health (1969). *Report on the confidential inquiries into maternal deaths in England and Wales for the years 1964-66* (HMSO).
Vaughan, Paul (1969) Family Planning, *The Family Planning Associa-tion Guide to Birth Control* (The Queen Anne Press, London).

3

Social Paediatrics

IT is the prayer of every parent, the desire of medicine and the hope of society, that foetal quality should be of the highest order. The intertwined aims of obstetrics and paediatrics endorse these ambitions. The discipline of obstetrics, as already described through antenatal care, interests itself in the care of the mother and infant. In former decades, the discipline of paediatrics commenced its interest in infant care on ligation of the umbilical cord. Now there are practitioners of foetal paediatrics, some of whom are deeply concerned with the development of the embryo. The science of human genetics has acquired a counselling role.

Each parent makes his or her genetical contribution to the hereditary endowment of the child. Characteristics which are present on the genotype do not necessarily show on the somotype. Some characteristics are modified by genetic mutation. Some are modified by environmental factors. Others are altered by a combination of both factors.

Factors such as childhood health of mother, nutrition and infection in pregnancy, hazards of the pre-, peri- and postnatal period all play a part in the early development of the child. The time-honoured forces of Nature and Nurture still and always will operate. Social factors such as occupation and income of father, housing conditions including overcrowding and ecology of the community are now being seen to have increasing influence.

The birth of an infant can be taken as a logical starting point for the delivery of health services. Initiation of the prime record is the foundation of the vital statistics. The former is the basis of the compulsory notification of birth to the medical officer of health within thirty-six hours of delivery, enforced in the United Kingdom since 1915. Registration of the birth of an infant in the United Kingdom must take place within forty-two days. Collation of this information provides the essential material for compilation of the birth-rate. An index of social progress in a community and the adequacy of health services is the declining number of infants who die before reaching their first birthday.

Infant Mortality Rate $= \dfrac{\text{Number of infants who die during the first year of life} \times 1000}{\text{Number of registered live births in that year}}$

In a developing community the deaths are spread over the first years. As advances in therapeutics and child care take their effect, the incidence of deaths from respiratory and alimentary infections is reduced, especially for infants between the age range of one to twelve months. Thus in civilized societies a finer guide in this field is required. So interest is concentrated on those infants who die during the first month of life, e.g. the neo-natal perod.

Neo-natal Mortality Rate $= \dfrac{\text{Number of infants who die during the first month of life} \times 1000}{\text{Number of registered live births in that year.}}$

In this time-span the majority of infants die during the first week of life.

Early Neo-natal Mortality Rate $= \dfrac{\text{Number of infants who die during the first week of life} \times 1000}{\text{Number of registered live births in that year.}}$

Since the majority of these infants involved at this early age die in the first few hours or days of life, it is logical to postulate that the factors involved in their deaths must be similar to those involved in infants who are born dead.

A stillbirth can be defined as any child which has issued forth from its mother after the 28th week of pregnancy and which did not at any time after being completely expelled from its mother breathe or show any other signs of life.

Stillbirth Rate $= \dfrac{\text{Number of stillbirths registered in one year} \times 1000}{\text{Total number of livebirths and stillbirths in that year}}$

Thus a more accurate term covering the late hazards of pregnancy and labour is the perinatal period.

Perinatal Mortality Rate $= \dfrac{\text{Total number of infants dying during the first week of life and the stillbirths registered during the year} \times 1000}{\text{Total number of livebirths and stillbirths registered during that year}}$

Detailed advances in obstetrics, paediatrics, and resuscitation have been concentrated in recent years on reducing this perinatal mortality rate. Prematurity, toxaemia, antepartum haemorrhage and congenital defects are the major causes of death. It should be pointed out that for the foreseeable future, there is a lower limit of possibly ten deaths per thousand live births and stillbirths, below which the perinatal mortality rate will not fall, since there are certain conditions involving prematurity and congenital malformation which are incompatible with life. As the infant mortality and perinatal mortality rates fall, certain infants, who would in former times have died, will thus survive and so increase the pool of handicapped children and adults. This truism must always be borne in mind: while the maternity services are reducing these infant death rates, the child health and education services will be gaining more complex human problems to solve.

Thus interlinked disciplines of medicine, genetics, psychology, education and sociology are all deeply involved in anticipating and detecting children with potential handicaps.

After correlating certain defects and handicaps with obstetric histories, the concept has been enunciated that certain infants, having passed through these hazards, are at special risk in showing these defects and handicaps. Thus 'at risk' or 'observation' registers can be compiled for these infants who are in need of detailed clinical surveillance. However, a clinical and academic debate is now current and validation is not yet firm, on the criteria of admission to an observation register. At first sight a short list of indications could be as follows:

1. History of parental deafness and/or dumbness.
2. Maternal viral infection during the first trimester, e.g. rubella.
3. Hydramnios and oligohydramnios.
4. Antepartum haemorrhage or threatened miscarriage.
5. Family history of congenital defect.
6. Prematurity—birth weight of 2494 g. or less.
7. Twin pregnancy.
8. Neo-natal asphyxia—a delay in establishing respiration.
9. Instrumental delivery or Caesarean section.
10. Neo-natal jaundice with a serum bilirubin level of say over 15 mg. per cent.
11. Failure to thrive.
12. Any other pre-, peri- or post-natal hazard.

However, if these and many other conditions are added, the
c

situation arises where an unmanageably high proportion of infants are added to the observation register.

A branch of medicine is now established whereby, in a detailed study of periodic careful clinical observation and examination, the development of the infant can be recorded from birth. Developmental screening of all infants and young children, with special attention to the 'at risk' groups, is held by a growing number of child health specialists to be the only way to detect and ameliorate handicaps and defects at their very earliest stage.

Particular attention is paid to responses to stimuli, neuromuscular co-ordination, special sensory abilities, special relationships. This branch of medicine is involved in the ascertainment and management of such conditions as congenital dislocation of the hip, cerebral palsy, infantile convulsions, disorders of communication, impaired mental endowment and social deprivation.

The screening should be conducted by personal physicians and child health doctors only after receiving training in these special skills. The detailed investigation after ascertainment of a deviation from normal development should be pursued at assessment centres within either a hospital or community health establishment by an integrated team of paediatricians, physiotherapists, psychologists and socio-medical workers, including those with a nursing background.

Congenital defects have a genetical basis to a greater or lesser extent, and the growing science of human genetics has a threefold responsibility in preventing the birth of handicapped children.

1. Where a handicapped child had been born into a family, the risk of further affected children being born to either the parents or the child's siblings could be accurately predicted.

2. Medical practitioners could be warned that a particular pregnancy was liable to produce a child with a hereditary defect.

3. As the techniques of treatment and testing advance, genetic counselling will ultimately lead to a marked reduction in the number of infants liable to inherit a serious mental or physical handicap. Parents could well be able to prevent the birth of an infant who either had, or might transmit, the defect concerned.

Considerable attention has been and is being paid to the physical well-being of the infant, and in recent decades emotional stability has also been recognized as being of increasing importance. The prime factor in the establishment of sound emotional infantile health is the creation of the mother/child relationship. If the nursing couple are not able to achieve a mutually satisfying attachment within six to eight weeks, then the risk of emotional deprivation is present. The motivation for the pregnancy may give a clue to such possible risk. Factors involved are:

1. Sibling rivalry.
2. Antagonism between mother and daughter.
3. The prevalence of morning sickness and behavioural problems in childhood.

Lack of early maternal affection in its severest form is considered by some to be a causal factor in childhood autism.

Infantile emotional development is dependent on the infant's basic equipment as to whether he has an out-turning or in-turning personality. In addition maturation of the infantile drives, aggression, and satisfaction of the hunger/feeding cycle, transition from milk to solid feeding, are involved. Failure to achieve results satisfying to both mother and infant can lead to frustrations and regression in the nursing couple relationship. Failure to thrive may be due to impaired mental endowment in the infant, but a strained emotional situation must be considered.

In the toddler age range, maternal understanding is required to support the child through his fears and fearfulness, jealousies of a newly arrived sibling, temper tantrums, social adaptations, and acceptance of toilet training. If the child is successful then his emotional stature is secure. Parental over-indulgence can be as damaging to an inadequate personality as lack of affection. The young child who achieves emotional stability during his first few years will be in a strong position to overcome the biological and emotional strains of adolescence.

The biological unit of the family is essential to a child's well-being and social development. Social deprivation with interlinked emotional and physical hazards can occur by:

(a) Famine, war.
(b) Death of one or both parents by illness or accident.
(c) Separation of the parents due to initial marriage break-up, divorce or imprisonment; or long-term in-patient hospital care of mother or child.

(d) One parent working excessively long hours or away from home.
(e) Inadequate personality of one parent.
(f) Unsupported mother.

The degree of deprivation is determined by:

1. Whether one or both parents is involved.
2. The amount of support given by one parent to the other.
3. Support given by relatives and neighbours.

Looking at the wider ecology of social deprivation there are three interlinked and interdependent forces:

1. *Medical.* The presence of mental illness, impaired mental endowment, emotional instability or physical handicap. The ready availability of the appropriate diagnosis and therapy determines the prognosis.
2. *Economic.* The opportunity to obtain a job in a given community with adequate wage to support a family varies both in time and place. Ill health impairs the wage earner's ability to either acquire or hold employment.
3. *Social.* The development and availability of social services to families with problems will vary with the economic health of the community concerned.

However, nearly every family, whatever its position in the economic and social scale of its society, has problems from time to time. A minority of these families with problems do not respond to any health or social measures in an adequate way and can be termed 'problem families'. Their characteristics include fecklessness, possible sexual promiscuity, inability to maintain relationships, and inability to organize their lives, with particular reference to the abstract.

The fundamental causation in the problem family is the inadequate personality, which is due in many instances to lack of emotional stability and parental affection in childhood. A vicious cycle can be postulated:

Problem family
↓
Deprived childhood
↓
Inadequate personality

The children of a problem family can be deprived of certain physical needs, while receiving a degree of emotional security. Society, through its services, in theory may wish to remove the children from these circumstances. The result will be emotionally deprived children and potential parents of a problem family in the next generation. Over the last two decades the social services, especially in the United Kingdom, have concentrated on supporting and maintaining these families together, in spite of all the difficulties that this policy encounters. The efficacy of these measures has still to be validated.

Social policy and child health measures are designed to ensure a childhood of optimum physical, emotional and social conditions.

REFERENCES

Alberman, E. D., Goldstein, H. (1970) The 'At-Risk' Register: A Statistical Evaluation. *British Journal of Preventive and Social Medicine*, 24, 129.

Bowlby, E. J. M. (1951) Maternal Care and Mental Health, WHO Monograph No. 2.

Carter, C. O. (1969) *An ABC of Medical Genetics (Lancet)*.

Egan, D. F., Illingworth, R. S., MacKeith, R. C. (1969) Developmental Screening 0–5 Years, *Clinics in Developmental Medicine* No. 30 (Heinemann Medical Books, London).

World Health Organisation (1967) The Early Detection and Treatment of Handicapped Defects in Young Children.

4

Detecting Disease and Disorder

THE disease process is determined by the underlying pathology.
The clinical features of a disease are demonstrated by:

1. Past and present history.
2. Symptoms described by the patient, e.g. pain, nausea, etc.
3. Signs ascertained by clinical examination and investigation.

Assessment of the clinical features and investigations, be they
bacteriological, histological, biochemical or radiological, will
define the differential diagnosis and finally the diagnosis of the
disease.

An individual may have noticed that he has certain signs and
symptoms, which are not too troublesome, such as a cough or
attacks of indigestion. He lives with these features and does not
seek medical aid. Self-medication may be administered. In due
course the individual decides that medical help should be sought;
he presents himself to his personal physician or the out-patient
department of a hospital. He is considered to be a patient, once he
requests medical therapy. The patient presents his disorder for
investigation and treatment. Medicine in many instances cannot
intervene, unless there is a readiness on the part of the individual
to request the skills of the discipline. Health and medical care
services handle only those patients who come forward with a disorder. It is like the tip of an iceberg. It is postulated that there
exists that portion of the clinical iceberg which is undetected and
unknown. A considerable number of individuals are aware of their
disorders, but have not been identified by the medical care services.
Thus a concept is enunciated that a high proportion of disorder
processes are known to the individual, but hidden from medicine.

In the pathological continuum of the disease process, the intervention of a histological or biochemical investigation would
ascertain the presence of that disease in an individual who was not
presenting signs and symptoms.

So certain clinical entities can be detected in a presymptomatic
stage. If a disease is identified in the presymptomatic stage it is

argued that early treatment will then supervene, with arrest and possible eradication of the pathology. It follows that if a population were subjected to specific screening procedures certain disease processes would be detected at an early stage and appropriate therapy initiated, and in certain instances the elimination of the complete disease could be achieved.

In relation to screening procedures, certain criteria have evolved, that:

1. The history and disease process is well understood.
2. The age group and likely victims can readily be identified.
3. The investigations involved are simple in application and acceptable to the individual and relatives.
4. Further intensive investigation (if required) and appropriate treatment are readily available with minimal time interval between primary identification and treatment.
5. The cost per case of identification is reasonable in relation to the health service resources.

Some diseases will attract these criteria on a hard basis, others at a given point of time will be considered to be softer.

Disease conditions with hard criteria

1. Congenital dislocation of the hip.
2. Metabolic disorders of infancy, e.g. phenylketonuria.
3. Infant deafness.
4. Pulmonary tuberculosis.
5. Anaemia, especially of the iron deficiency type.
6. Carcinoma of the cervix.

Moderate criteria.

7. Diabetes.
8. Breast and lung cancer.
9. Hypertension.
10. Urinary infection.
11. Venereal disease.
12. Visual defects.
13. Psychiatric disorders.

Soft criteria.

14. Chronic bronchitis.
15. Glaucoma.

With the advance of medical knowledge and technology diseases will move from one category to another. Other diseases will be added. Pilot epidemiological studies and surveys are required to determine those diseases which meet the criteria already determined.

Opinion is hardening that the value of population screening as a national policy in the majority of disease instances so enunciated be considered, to use a Scottish judicial term, as non proven. However, the grand strategy of medicine is moving towards the postulation that whenever a medical check, assessment and examination is undertaken, then proven screening procedures should be incorporated. Well-designed history questionnaires in conjunction with automated pathological techniques, sound and detailed clinical examination, humane and sympathetic counselling, lead to a fruitful, balanced medical check situation.

Health services should be so structured that individuals, irrespective of age and sex, can present themselves for such medical checks. In addition, whenever a patient seeks medical advice, a detailed socio-medical ascertainment should be made. Common sense supervenes in that repeated medical screening situations at decreasing time intervals could be considered ridiculous, if carried out with ruthless efficiency and misguided enthusiasm.

A logical approach in the design of health services to create such a medical screening situation can be based on an age/sex structure.

1. *Infant*

(a) As previously indicated, periodic developmental medical examinations can be carried out. Every infant, prior to being discharged from hospital, should receive a complete detailed neurological examination by a paediatric specialist in developmental medicine. Thereafter periodic examinations by child health doctors should be made at six weeks, three, six, nine, twelve and eighteen months and yearly thereafter. Included in these examinations would be a clinical test for dislocation of the hip, and hearing assessment.

It could be argued, at this point of time, that there are

insufficient doctors trained in this type of medicine to undertake such an ideal programme. Attention must be paid to the
vocational training of child health specialists and of all
doctors who examine and see infants on a routine basis. As
an interim measure, the use of questionnaire techniques
involving the mother, or other socio-medical workers
(especially those with a nursing background), may well be
indicated.

Any infant with a deviation from normal development,
which may be due to interdependent physical, mental,
emotional and social factors, should be sent to an assessment
centre for full investigation, in sophisticated and well
organized communities where these exist.

(b) Metabolic disorders. All infants, whether born in hospital or
in the community, should be screened by either a urine or
blood investigation at the earliest age indicated. Blood
samples depending on chromatography (Guthrie and
Scrivers tests) are taking the place of the cruder urine
investigation. Positive results call for full biochemical investigation.

Close collaboration is essential between the hospital and
community-based health services to ensure that no infant is
missed.

2. Pre-school Child

There is a difference in terminology for the age group two
to five years. The time honoured term 'toddler' persists, but
a rampaging three-year-old makes nonsense of such a
definition. 'Pre-school child' is probably more descriptive.
Children in this age group require a detailed clinical examination involving all systems. A complete history will determine
previous episodes of illness. Failure to reach acceptable
norms or milestones of development must be looked into
further. Particular attention should be paid to emotional
stability, including socialization, the ability to communicate
and the response to stimuli. Examination of urine for sub-
acute infection, and faeces for infestation is ideal if laboratory
facilities are available.

Children with a defect must be kept under close surveillance. If the defect is minor, steps must be taken to

ensure that it does not worsen. If due to untoward circumstances the defect is severe, appropriate treatment, including
special educational and social therapy, can be instituted.

3. *School Child*

(a) In many communities and societies the young child enters a
nursery school at two or three years, with transfer to more
formal education at five to six years. The timing of the first
routine periodic medical inspection can be either prior to or
after school entry. There are advantages and disadvantages
in the timing, but whatever method is adopted the alerting
of the parent and teacher, by appropriate medical advice, to
any deviation from normal is essential.

A history from the parent involving previous infectious
illnesses and immunization state is essential. Again, a full
clinical examination is required with particular attention to
cardiac, orthopaedic, and upper respiratory defects. Prior
to such a periodic medical inspection, the results of hearing
and vision testing and urinary screening should be made
available to the examining doctor for the school. Defects may
either be:

(i) Kept under surveillance and reviewed at regular intervals.
(ii) Treated through the appropriate curative service.

A school health service, based on historic orthodox lines,
will endeavour to carry out three or four routine periodic
medical inspections during the child's life: at school entry
(5–6 years), at transition (7–8 years), at transfer from junior
to secondary education (10–11 years) and prior to leaving
school (13 years plus). This programme involves a heavy
load on medical manpower and alternative methods to
ensure greater depth in medical consultation have been
sought. It is agreed, in the present state of our knowledge,
that the school entry and leaving routine periodic medical
inspections should be retained.

If the intermediate inspections are dropped, the following
screening procedures should be substituted:

(i) Questionnaires into health and educational progress,
completed by parent and teacher respectively, for

scrutiny by an experienced school doctor for significant answers. A clinical examination should be carried out in appropriately selected cases. For example, failure to make educational progress may be due to impaired mental endowment, incipient behavioural difficulties, or defective vision or hearing.

(ii) Screening for visual and hearing defects using appropriate vision screening apparatus and audiometers. The ancillary staff used would refer 'failured' cases for further medical inquiry.

The medical inspection prior to leaving school has the twofold purpose of remedying any defect and advising of the medical aspects of vocational guidance.

(b) *Special examinations.* Parents and teachers must have the right to approach the school health service for further investigation and advice if they are concerned about a particular child's health and educational progress.

(c) *Dental Surveillance.* An integral part of a school health service is the school dental service. Routine dental inspections should be conducted on an annual basis if possible. Appropriate treatment—either conservative, orthodontic, or radical —should be completed for dental pathology and deviations.

(d) *Miscellaneous Surveillance.* Educational systems need built-in psychological advice and expertise. The educational psychologist, in collaboration with teachers, seeks out, tests and investigates those children who have learning difficulties, e.g. retarded reading. Remedial teaching can be invaluable. However, as previously indicated, failure to make educational progress has a multifactorial causation requiring a team approach, including medical opinion.

Speech therapists, in association with teachers, conduct surveys in school. Thus children with speech difficulties can either be kept under surveillance, receive therapy, or be referred for further investigation. Orthopaedic defects can be sought out in the same way by appropriately trained staff.

Hygiene inspections by nursing personnel at least every three months will detect head and body lice, skin infections (impetigo, scabies, ringworm and plantar warts). In civilized countries injection marks should also be sought for drug experimentation.

Physical education and swimming bath instructors can be shown contagious skin lesions, and their inspections prior to the physical activity concerned will screen these out and aid epidemiological control. This procedure may not at first sight be acceptable to all medical practitioners, but with careful instruction from the physician responsible for epidemiology, early detection of troublesome lesions leads to earlier and effective treatment of the individual school child.

4. *Young Person*

The age range could be defined as the period from the teens to the twenties. There is an overlap, depending on maturity, with the schoolchild and with the adult.

The routine medical inspection for the school leaver prior to entering an occupation, employment or craft, has already been mentioned. An epidemiological and preventive tool, which is also a screening procedure, is the testing of children for sensitivity to tuberculosis by using tuberculin from the age of twelve years. Some authorities believe that the earlier age of ten to eleven years is more appropriate.

A small dose of tuberculin is either injected subcutaneously or by multiple puncture technique into the skin of the forearm. The test is read seventy-two hours later.

Result of reading:

(a) If reaction is within a predetermined criterion, then a positive reaction is recorded. The significance being that the individual young person has a degree of immunity to tuberculosis from previous exposure and likely infection. The individual should be clinically investigated, including radiological examination of the chest. If necessary, the immediate family contacts should also be screened. In this way those suffering from pulmonary tuberculosis can be detected, treated and brought under surveillance.

(b) If there is no dermatological response, then a negative reaction is recorded. The individual is offered protection by vaccination with BCG (Bacillus of Calmette and Guérin) at once. A sample (ten per cent) of the vaccinated persons should be retested with tuberculin at a later date to ascertain the degree and efficiency of conversion. A high conversion rate is to be expected.

Young persons entering particular callings, such as nurses and medical students, who may be exposed to undiagnosed sufferers from pulmonary tuberculosis, should receive such screening.

A routine medical examination for young people entering industry and commerce is carried out in a systematic way by many enlightened employers, in some communities as a legal requirement. However, these inspections are not as widespread and as detailed as is desirable. In establishments of higher education, both universities and technical colleges, student health services are growing in importance. Although medical examination and radiological examination of the chest may not be mandatory, firm advice is given and accepted by students on their initial matriculation.

In summary, further study and evaluation is required to detect emotional and other disease processes for many young people who at present are not covered by any specific health care service.

5. *The Adult*

Recruits for the armed and emergency services and candidates for insurance policies, have been subjected to clinical examination and medical questionnaires. Entry to certain occupations, appointments and callings has demanded either a medical examination or assessment, including radiological examination of the chest. The main purpose is to determine the likelihood and frequency of absence due to sickness, even of a minor nature. A secondary purpose is an actuarial one of forecasting the reliability of a contributor to a superannuation scheme. This latter requirement is not as important as the former. Medical opinion is forming that a clinical examination is not absolutely necessary in this regard, and that a selective health questionnaire is all that is required. A significant history would entail a clinical assessment in great depth. These procedures would detect disease and disorder, and appropriate advice as to the matching of the individual to his occupation would ensue. Applicants for driving licences in many communities are called upon to give a health history or to be medically examined. Certain bar diseases, such as uncontrolled epilepsy, subnormality and attacks of giddiness, may come to light, safeguarding the individual and the community as a whole. Drivers of public service vehicles and heavy lorries have special responsibilities and are subject to specific medical requirements.

As previously indicated, the philosophy and purpose of antenatal care provides a medical check situation with built-in screening procedures: the examination of the urine; blood pressure tests; blood investigations for anaemia, syphilis, and gonorrhoea; blood grouping, including the Rh. factor; chest X-ray; height and weight estimations, and the care of the foetus. The resultant postnatal examination is vital as a preventive gynaecological screening technique: position and health of cervix and uterus; state of uterine and vaginal walls; presence of vaginal discharge; general state of health, and where appropriate, advice on birth control.

Women who have families are familiar with these two essential medical care programmes. If they seek contraceptive advice from their personal medical adviser, or agency specializing in this field, a full clinical, including gynaecological and cytological, investigation of the cervix is carried out. All clinical entities are corrected or treated.

If a smear from the cervix of the uterus is subjected to cytological examination, cells of

(a) Pre-cancerous state (cancer *in situ*)
(b) Invasive cancer cells

can be detected. Smears from the vagina can be obtained at the same time. Based on this pathological technique, comprehensive population screening of women has taken place all over the world, the duration of some covering nearly two decades. The critical test of such expenditure in time, money, and resources is a marked reduction in the number of deaths due to carcinoma of the cervix. An academic debate on the preliminary results has been joined. Evaluation and validation are being assessed with considerable statistical and intellectual vigour. A recall of every three years is desirable from a negative test result. Every woman who presents herself for a vaginal examination should have this smear taken as part of the spectrum of required investigations.

In order to build in the screening procedure of cervical cytology, some health services and personal doctors organize 'well women' clinics for a full clinical examination and counselling. Such procedures include:

Blood examination for anaemia.
Urine tests—including those for subclinical infection.
Examination of breast—and instruction in self-examination.
Radiological examination of chest.
Contraceptive advice and therapy if required.
Gynaecological examination and counselling.

Thus physical, emotional, psycho-sexual deviations and aberrations can be screened and appropriate therapy initiated.

It could be argued that there is a place for 'well men' clinics. Business and commercial enterprises in sophisticated societies are encouraging their higher executives to undergo medical checks. A full history and clinical examination is required. The lower age range should be thirty to thirty-five years. This style of medical check is still in its very early stages of development.

After the age of fifty-five, the role of the medical check prior to retirement and to cover the elderly is becoming firmly established. The range of clinical, biochemical and histological investigations is as wide as those included for younger adults. Nutritional advice is paramount. The inclusion of a mental health specialist in the team is invaluable in screening out the emotional and psycho-sexual deviations.

In conclusion, while population screening surveys must be undertaken to validate their criteria, a more worthwhile strategy is the inclusion of these procedures in the medical check situation.

REFERENCES

Medical Commission on Accident Prevention. *Fitness to Drive* (1968).
Screening in Medical Care, Nuffield Provincial Hospitals Trust (Oxford University Press, 1968).
Wilson, J. M. G., Jungner, G. (1968). Principles and Practice of Screening for Disease, *Public Health Papers 34*, WHO.

5

Vulnerable Groups

THE provision of health services is often all-embracing in its approach and, allied with the overall strategy of the presymptomatic diagnosis of disease, a blanket cover effect results. To ensure the economic use of health service resources both in money and personnel in all types of society, the detection and support of groups vulnerable to physical, mental, and social forces is becoming a philosophy of significant interest. The diagnosis and therapy for these groups involves the interface between the disciplines of medicine, sociology and psychology. Students and practitioners of these disciplines must appreciate that no one discipline is predominant at all times, but all are dependent on each other. It is becoming accepted that the detection of the physically, emotionally and socially weak is a prudent line of social policy and political action. Reference has already been made in an indirect way to some of the vulnerable groups, and a degree of minimal overlap cannot be avoided. Age and sex factors provide a basic structure. It could be argued that programmes involving the medical check situation, with screening procedures, should concentrate on these vulnerable groups because the return for effort and resource would be optimal. Time and experience will confirm this line of reasoning.

A starting point in this consideration is marriage, which is the most complex human relationship any individual is called upon to enter. An enrichment of character, personality, and well-being comes to the majority of married couples, and even to some stable cohabitors. However, to a minority marital harmony is not achieved with the first partner nor with subsequent partners. An inadequate personality, under stress in certain cultures, may feel that marriage offers an escape from social pressures. There are two chances for the resultant union. If the other partner is of strong character and personality, resourceful, understanding and responsible, the weaker partner will gain solace and even maturity. The second chance is that if both partners are inadequate, the relationship in marriage will be biologically shaky from its commencement. Stress in a physical, emotional or social form may recur and breakdown can ensue.

The historical practice of the marriage prearranged by parents, based on economic stability, exists in many societies throughout the world. This axiom of society stability is being replaced by individuals seeking out their own mates. Rivalry between siblings, especially sisters, drives certain women into marriage. Antagonism between mother and daughter may have the same effect in the younger woman's hastened dive into matrimony.

In certain primitive, especially agricultural, communities, young couples are not discouraged by their elders from practising sexual intercourse. Pregnancy means that the subsequent marriage will be fruitful, and is therefore blessed. Fertility is sacrosanct in that extra pairs of hands are the best biological investment for the future.

In other societies pre-marital intercourse is not formally recognized and a forced or 'shotgun' marriage is performed, so that society accepts the subsequent pregnancy and infant within its moral and legal code. Thus a relationship which was primarily a biological experiment and experience may result in unhappy legal bondage. The couple presenting at the altar as a threesome often, in civilized countries, start their connubial home with one or other set of parents. The latter may superficially welcome the couple, but deeply resent the circumstances. A husband in his wife's parents' house may be the subject of deep anger in that he is possibly guilty of having deflowered their daughter. The converse is also apparent, in that a wife in her husband's parents' household, may be denigrated in that she seduced their son. These attitudes can exist, even if the couple do not join a parental household. Whatever the circumstances, strained family dynamics exist, which are fraught with disharmony. Tensions build up which strike at the basis of stable emotional family life, and the social therapy of fresh housing accommodation may well be imperative.

Rather than enter into the legal and moral strait-jacket of a forced or shotgun marriage, couples armed with contraceptive knowledge and expertise attempt to establish stable cohabitation relationships or 'trial marriages', the reasoning being that if the trial is successful then legal marriage can be contemplated with confidence. Emotional and social strains result from fear that the fragile bond, based on mutual trust and confidence, will be snapped by one or other partner walking out. The resultant emotional and

D

mental trauma can be deep. A fear of pregnancy exists if there is forgetfulness or carelessness in the contraceptive technique.

With the advent of oral contraceptives the responsibility for a pregnancy has passed to the female. If a couple, in their love play, are bent on sexual intercourse, the man asks the woman if she is taking 'The Pill' and if the answer is in the affirmative, then the man is assured and may dispense with the male contraceptive precautions. In fact, if her answer is untrue and the woman is not taking her oral contraceptive, a pregnancy can result. The man has been seduced and trapped into marriage or dependent relationship. The male is now vulnerable as a result of a modern contraceptive advance.

Pregnancy can be used as an escape from reality, both within and outside marriage. The pregnant woman feels that she will be nurtured and cared for by her consort, husband and society. Exposure to the risk of pregnancy, especially in the unmarried and separated, may give rise to pseudo symptoms of conception, e.g. amenorrhoea, nausea, and attacks of giddiness. If further clinical examination and investigation do not confirm the pregnancy, the individual has anyway received say six to eight weeks of sympathetic attention and care. When the diagnosis is not confirmed, support and counselling is very necessary, in addition to contraceptive advice.

Attention has already been drawn to the vulnerability existing after an abortion or stillbirth. The urge to become pregnant may have deep and complex motivations. If this desire is constantly expressed, professional advisers should be on the alert, since the outcome for any child may be none too secure. Adoption may be contemplated by a neurotic wife to save a shaky marriage; this suggestion may have been made by professional advisers. Adoption should never be advised under these circumstances, since the welfare of the infant is of prime concern.

The majority of pregnant women are young and healthy and produce normal lusty infants. There is, however, an instinctive fear of labour, with the possibility that an abnormal infant will be born. Mothercraft and psychoprophylaxis help to alleviate and overcome these fears. If on sound clinical grounds, anaesthetic or operative intervention is indicated, the mother may feel that she has been a failure in that she was not able to deliver herself with minimal aid, as she had been led to expect by previous teaching. The professional attendants may not always accept and understand relaxation techniques. An awkward and derisory attitude is adopted, with the resultant feeling of failure by the mother. Where a high proportion of deliveries take place in hospital, the through-put is rapid and turnover is high. The midwifery and medical staff become overworked. There is risk of a humane, comforting approach being lost. There is no time to understand and allay the mother's fears. The relationship between mother and professional staff is strained, and a lack of confidence and a feeling of rejection results. The new mother at her most vulnerable is lost and fearful. She may then decide that taking her own discharge home against professional advice and on her own responsibility is the only course open to her. Her advisers in the community, on her return home, are faced with a mother whose self-confidence is shattered, and in need of tremendous support and help. Fortunately these circum-stances do not occur frequently, but those who are interested in community health must not forget them.

Reference has already been made to the factors of risk which require an infant to be placed on an observation register. The advent of an infant with a physical or mental defect evokes a varying degree of parental emotional response. The spread of reaction can be from over-protection to frank rejection. The feeling of guilt is present. The manner in which the diagnosis, care, therapy, and prognosis is conveyed to the parents requires all the expertise and understanding possessed by the doctor con-cerned. The primary interview, when this distressing disclosure is made, may give the professional adviser the impression that his observations have been calmly received. The original emotional trauma is often cloaked by numbness but the subsequent feelings of guilt are inevitable. The numbness fades after a time and the true basic reaction comes through.

These vulnerable parents must be supported and counselled. The listening ear must be available. Separation of the handicapped infant from his parents into a hospital or special residential unit may be indicated, to allow the parents time to adjust to the new situation. Other parents may feel that they must care for this handicapped infant from the outset and to the limits of their health and strength. However, the roles of assessment units, child health doctors and community nurses must be readily available to support, counsel and guide the parents over their very real emotional and physical problems.

The unsupported mother and her baby are a single-parent

family. If she marries or returns to her relatives, or enters into a stable cohabiting relationship, a completely or partially secure background for the child may be established. However, the decision at delivery, which can be heart-rending is whether the unsupported mother should keep the baby with her and rear it herself, or submit it for adoption. A temporary expedient would be for the infant to be cared for by others, by either private fostering or formal child care services. The expectant mother, if unmarried, may indicate in pregnancy that she wishes the infant to be adopted at the due time. When she sees and cuddles her own infant, a very strong emotional bond of affection is aroused. She revokes her previous decision and wishes to keep the child. Over the neonatal period and beyond, her mind is wrestling with the decision. In some maternity units, if there is a possibility of the infant's being adopted, the child is parted from the mother at birth, so that the bonds of knowledge and affection are never established. This practice would appear to be cruel, since the mother will suffer emotionally from the 'empty arms' syndrome, as in the post-stillbirth period. Whether the infant stays with its mother or not, the initial decision to let the formal adoption proceedings be initiated should not take place until the infant is six weeks old. In many societies the pressure to have the infant adopted comes from the maternal grandparents, who are fearful of the ridicule and disgrace. Other grandparents, if their own daughter is young, may rear the child as their own.

However, many are moving towards a more flexible and liberal attitude towards the unsupported mother and her child by better child care and welfare services, and the dropping of punitive attitudes. More unsupported mothers are attempting to keep their infants and make a home for them. If they have been rendered homeless and have left their own families, special provisions are required. If shelter is acquired, the mother will need to work, and day care for the infant is necessary. The appropriate social therapy can be:

1. Child Minding. The mother places the child in the care of another, not a relative, for reward. In England and Wales child minders are registered and inspected by local authority officers.
2. Private day nursery staffed by duly qualified persons where the daily or weekly charge is set by the proprietor.

3. Day nursery organized by the local authority where the daily or weekly charge is determined after due assessment of the mother's financial resources and commitments.

In England and Wales the day nurseries have priority groups for admission. Voluntary societies are now establishing houses in multiple occupation, or flatlets. Enlightened housing authorities are accepting these single-parent families as applicants on the housing waiting list.

If day care cannot be arranged, or breaks down, the mother may feel that her child should leave her for a while until times are better. Then overnight as well as day care is brought into effect.

1. *Fostering.* The mother places the child in another person's home. In England and Wales:

(a) If the individual fosters children for under twenty-eight days, then no registration with the local authority is necessary.
(b) If the individual fosters children for over twenty-eight days, then registration and inspection by the local authority is necessary. Any charge is a private arrangement between the mother and the foster parent.

2. *Residential nursery.* Voluntary societies administer such establishments. The mother makes application to the society for admission of her child. These units are registered and inspected.

3. *Local authorities.* Local Authorities in England and Wales can take the child into care and have alternative arrangements:
(a) Boarding out. Certain individuals receive a weekly remuneration from the local authority for receiving children into their homes. Such fostering can be on either a short or long term basis.
(b) Residential nursery.

Reference has already been made to the undesirable policy of separating mother and child. Every effort is made by financial and social work support to keep mother and child together. However, complex circumstances may force separation.

The sudden death of an infant is a shattering episode for the parents, relatives, and professional advisers. A 'cot death' can be due either to inhalation of vomit, milk allergy, acute respiratory infection or suffocation due to plastic covered pillows and mattresses. Suffocation is the most frequent cause of accidental death in infants under one.

In the toddler, who is an inquisitive character, burns, lacerations, crushed fingers and poisoning are the commonest accidents. Some young children are neglected by parents who have impaired mental endowment. For example, the child scalded in a bath of hot water which was not tested prior to immersion. These families are often known to social welfare services, relatives, and neighbours. In a minority group, wilful neglect and violence of repeated attacks has to be recognized. A subtle universal syndrome of the abused child is being recognized including the 'battered baby'. The child is subjected to attack with resultant injury. There is delay in seeking medical aid and the history is dubious. The story does not tally with the combined features of the siting and severity of the injuries and the alleged circumstances. All medical care services who see children with injuries, however minor, should be alert to such a possibility, when the factors just indicated are present.

The predisposing factors are:

1. History of violence, especially in the father.
2. Unemployment or frequent job changes.
3. Inadequate personality of one or both parents, including rejection of child.
4. Mother's pregnancy at time of episode.
5. The father of child is not necessarily the husband.
6. Social isolation: family has had frequent moves from one area to another.

Although the ascertainment of this syndrome is difficult and its true incidence is not accurately known, social welfare and medical care services, psychiatric, contraceptive, and paediatric help must Be given by the medical care services in collaboration with social welfare disciplines. Court action may have to be initiated on account of the severity of injury.

A pre-school child needs the freedom of space, fresh air, opportunity to play with his peers and to make a noise. It follows that when and where these freedoms are restricted, the child is vulnerable and at risk as far as physical, emotional and social development are concerned. Society in advanced civilizations advocates and orranges day care facilities, often with an educational bias. It is to be regretted that a high proportion of children in the world are

hungry and socially deprived, and receive either no formal education, or only in a very limited form. This estimate has been put as
high as eighty per cent of total world child population.

The child, on school entry, has to adjust and adapt to a more
formal régime. Reactions may present themselves as reluctance to
attend, refusal to eat, impaired educational progress or frequent
sick absence on limited clinical grounds.

The child with a physical, emotional or mental defect can, with
support and understanding, be absorbed into the normal educational system. If the child is handicapped to such a degree that this
absorption is not possible, then arrangements must be made for
special educational treatment. An earlier age for the commencement of this educational therapy than the age of formal school
entry may be desirable or essential.

These handicaps can be multiple, with one particular handicap
predominant. The spectrum of handicaps where special educational treatment is indicated are as follows: blindness, partial sight,
deafness, impaired hearing, physical disabilities (e.g. cerebral
palsy, hydrocephalus and *spina bifida*), defective speech, epilepsy,
impaired mental endowment, behavioural difficulties and emotional maladjustment, delicacy (e.g. asthma and general debility).
The educational treatment can take a number of forms:

1. Modification of education in an ordinary school, e.g. special
   transport arrangements. For instance a child with impaired
   hearing sits with the good ear near the teacher.
2. Special class in an ordinary school. A group of handicapped
   pupils at the same educational level of ability are given
   tuition together.
3. Special schools, on either a day or residential basis. This
   facility is determined by incidence of given handicap in
   population, geography and transport arrangements.
4. Hospital school.

In general terms it is accepted that blind and deaf handicapped
pupils must attend a special school, so that sophisticated educational methods and techniques can be used. With other handicaps
ingenuity, understanding, and good will may make special school
placement unnecessary.

The child who fails to make educational progress is vulnerable
and needs remedial help and investigation. Possible causes of this
delay are:

1. Impaired mental endowment, especially if mental age is two years or more below the chronological age.
2. Visual or hearing impairment calling for correction by appropriate aids.
3. Emotional and behavioural difficulties. The child appears to be developing normally in school, but progress in, say, reading and number work is retarded. The answer could well be at home in the social circumstances or strained family dynamics. The emotional difficulties showing in a somatic form, e.g. bed-wetting.
4. Frequent sick absence or long duration of illness; and truancy.

Attention has been paid to the one-parent family in its formation, when an infant is born to an unsupported mother. A two-parent family can become a one-parent family on:

1. Death of parent, especially the father.
2. Separation of parents: break-up of marriage, or imprisonment of one parent.
3. Illness, with long spell of in-patient hospital care for one or other parent.
4. One or other parent becoming physically or mentally handicapped, and enabled to live at home but not to work.

The children of these families are at risk of being socially deprived. The remaining parent, of economic necessity, has to work. There is debate as to whether in a two-parent family where the father works, the mother should also seek, obtain and pursue employment outside or inside the home. The obvious advantage is that the mother brings in an additional wage or income. She is able to follow a profession or occupation for which she is trained and is a more confident and satisfied individual. The disadvantage is that a young child does not receive full-time affection from his mother, since substitute day care will be used. If a school child falls sick, he is deprived because his mother is not able to give him all the attention she might. It should be pointed out that certain women do not care for child rearing, they feel the need to go out to work, and use their homes only as a base.

The period of adolescence can be a smooth biological transition from childhood to adulthood. There is a conflict between the urge to be emancipated as an individual in one's own right and the need for reassurance and support. The young want to be liked and accepted by their equals. Their relationship with their parents undergoes a change from one of dependence to one of equality. This adjustment can set up disillusionment and antagonism. The vast majority of parents and their adolescent offspring reach a more mature and satisfying relationship. A minority do not do so. Parents, even though incompatible and with their marriage biologically disintegrating, decide to live together 'for the sake of the children'. The father does not match up to his daughter's ideal as a man. The mother is over-protective towards her son. The latter quarrels with his father, the daughter does not 'get on' with her mother. The young, developing individuals seek other relationships and outlets. Misdemeanours against society are committed, including petty larceny, truancy, violence against persons and property, especially in the tribe or gang complex. This disharmony with the social code is a clue to individuals in need of help. An inadequate personality under stress may leave home, wander, and fall in with like-thinking spirits, who may 'drop out' from society. If the culture is a drug-taking one, then the condition of dependence on soft or hard drugs is established.

Youth throughout the world, irrespective of creed or colour, is questioning the structure of society. If dissatisfaction is felt then this 'drop-out' syndrome occurs. Adolescents are susceptible to sexual misadventure, in that they are involved and wish to explore their own sexuality. They are interested in forming biological relationships with members of the opposite sex. They both fear and are intrigued by sexuality. They wish to explore the boundaries of human relations. Those individuals who are stable personalities, and are knowledgeable in human relations in all its aspects, have no serious difficulties. Others, however, become involved in serious emotional tangles, including the physiological end result—pregnancy.

The young person on leaving school enters an occupation, craft, or vocation. Additional attendance at establishments of higher education is often a basic requirement to achieve appropriate qualifications. Individuals who frequently change jobs and cannot keep them for any length of time are those who fail to achieve job satisfaction. Their personalities and/or emotional instability may be responsible. By the same token the examination failure, especially the persistent one, is in need of help. Mental illness must always be borne in mind. Special attention must be paid to the handicapped school leaver, who needs considerable vocational guidance and help.

This narrative started with marriage and has described the risk areas for the infant and indirectly for the marriage partners. The young mother is concerned about her ability to manage and care for a young growing family. Her husband, unless crippled by accident, especially head injury, strives to earn an economic wage or salary to support the family. The prime ambition is to acquire adequate housing. In the balancing of priorities for distribution of the family economic resources, in times of stress, payment of rent is deferred. Among the causes of homelessness, repeated rent arrears is high. Therefore in the detection of the family with problems, a poor rent payment record is a shrewd indicator.

The young married man in his late twenties and early thirties, especially if he is in the executive grades, is striving with tremendous vigour to establish himself. The competition is keen. He tends to eat, smoke and drink too much, and not take enough exercise. He may be travelling by air around the world on business trips. His time with his wife and family is limited. Family tensions are set up and decision-making between the partners is either postponed or taken unilaterally. Such an individual may shun his family and seek outside interests other than work, for example alcohol or gambling. The latter pursuits may be at a social level, but the transition to compulsive allegiance is very short and narrow. Certain habits and physical disorders can be detected in this group:

1. Overeating and overweight.
2. Raised blood pressure.
3. Heavy smoking and alcohol consumption.
4. Inadequate exercise.
5. Early diabetes.

These men are candidates for coronary occlusive attacks, which can be fatal.

Death or incapacity of the main breadwinner is a major family disaster and a severe loss of educational investment as far as society is concerned. It follows that more attention must be paid to the health and well-being of young and middle-aged men, since their burden of social and economic responsibility is high.

When the youngest child of the family has left school or home, the parents have to adjust to this new situation. The composition of the family may be such that young grandchildren are about. If the family has been a small one this situation may not arise, or not for a little time. The mother, may have little to occupy her time. She may be able to undertake a job on either a whole or part time basis, or else she may have sufficient hobbies and interests to satisfy her needs. Otherwise the effects of loneliness will set in. Social welfare services should be aware of these circumstances and preparation for retirement is appropriate.

The acquisition of hobbies and interests should really start in childhood, however, the early fifties is not too late to take up leisure pursuits. In addition pre-retirement courses for older people at establishments of further education include such subjects as nutrition, home economics, house purchase, etc. There is sometimes a desire on the part of older people on retirement to move to more salubrious surroundings, often by the seaside. Without adequate and careful preparation over a period of years such moves may end in loneliness and despair. As civilization advances and age expectancy increases, an acceptable mean age of retirement is sixty-five years. A new set of circumstances are arising in that couples in their late sixties and early seventies still have the responsibility of their older relatives in the late eighties and nineties. One can postulate a new work pattern in that:

1. An individual receives his education and initial training for a craft in his late teens.
2. (a) That craft or skill will no longer be necessary and the individual needs retraining in the early thirties.
   or (b) primary training in the calling is reached by late twenties or thirties and an intensive period of executive responsibility lasts until the early fifties.
3. Further adaptation of skills to operate at a slower pace could be indicated from the mid-fifties so that the individual would not block promotion, but work on until the early seventies.

Older people need adequate preparation for retirement and if an orderly way of life is followed, with good health, a happy revered existence is assured. However, this rosy picture can be besmirched if:

(a) The death of a marriage partner, close relative, or friend takes place. The first three weeks are very important to ensure that the individual has adequate nourishment, since there is a marked reluctance to eat. Then further social welfare support and counselling is required.

(b) There are disorders of locomotion and other crippling conditions. If older persons cannot get out of their homes on account of crippled feet, arthritis of the lower limbs, or severe cardiac and respiratory embarrassment, then loneliness can supervene. Social contact with the community outside is lost.

(c) There is loneliness for other reasons. This social disease has a variety of causes. Movement from one community to another will bring on social isolation, unless steps are taken to avoid it. The elderly are more prone to this condition than are younger people. Once an individual starts to lose social contact, there is a marked reluctance towards re-establishment. Lack of social contact deteriorates into severe social isolation.

A final area of vulnerability is the movement of individuals and families from the country of their own ethnic culture to a country of alien culture. The adoption and absorption of one culture by another is a very slow, tedious process. The differences in health practices, feeding patterns, clothing styles and religious customs, are a subject in themselves. However, education, health, and social welfare services, including housing, may be left to solve the problems, if they do not have to cope with too many individuals at any one time.

REFERENCES

National Society for Mentally Handicapped Children (1967) *Stress in Families with a Mentally Handicapped Child.*

Torrie, M., *Begin Again* (Dent, 1970).

Younghusband, E. (1970) *Living with Handicap.* National Bureau for Cooperation in Child Care.

6

Diseases of Society and their Therapy

REFERENCE will be made to the control of infectious diseases.
The community has established standards and controls to prevent
their spread. There are other non-infectious clinical entities which
have a sociological origin and an epidemiology of their own. In many
instances, observers of medicine in the community are firmly con-
vinced that if the individual patient had had basic health information these diseases might never have flourished. A more complex
situation arises when the individual, having this health knowledge,
fails to take advantage of it. Possession of health knowledge, rather
than acting as a deterrent, may act as a stimulant to experiment.
On balance, knowledge of health, in the long term, is for the good
of the individual and the community as a whole, rather than having
any short-term deleterious effect. Thus the philosophy and strategy
of health education programmes must be evaluated over one or
more decades, rather than weeks, months or years.

Parents have the prime responsibility of educating their children
in health matters over a long period of time by a process of absorption, so that when they in their turn become parents, they will
have the basic knowledge to pass on to their own children. However,
in the second half of the twentieth century, the majority of parents
do not have this knowledge of health. Even those who do possess
this information and experience are faced with a problem of communication in simple terms. Much of the descriptive terminology
is derived from the ancient classical languages. Other terms can be
in the crude, earthy vernacular of the community concerned.
Therefore the communicators of this health knowledge have to
present it to all ages in a form that can be understood, accepted,
assimilated and acted upon. The parameters and areas of health
education overlap and have been mentioned elsewhere.

Human relationships are a fundamental area of knowledge, with
the accent on the responsibility for oneself and one's actions and
other human beings. At first sight simple anatomy and physiology
of both the plant and animal kingdoms can be absorbed by young
children. More detailed structure and functions can be assimilated,

45

with particular reference to the genito-urinary tract, including the menstrual cycle for young girls. Then the more complex subjects of conception, foetal growth, delivery and infant care. Finally, emotional relationships, including love and responsibility, promiscuity and venereal disease. The qualifications of the health educator in this field, while of importance, need not be confined to one discipline. The ability to teach, combined with a flexible, understanding personality, is of prime importance. The biology teacher, with the support of health visitor and medical practitioner, would form a suitable team. For older schoolchildren, it is argued that if they had a knowledge of contraception then the social consequences of unwanted children, illegitimacy and abortion would be avoided. A more positive approach to human relationships with responsibility, especially in the man, is the aim.

Within every country in the world, be it advanced or developing, there are many individuals who have an imbalance of diet in regard to both quality and quantity. In some countries the proportion of the mal- and under-nourished individuals is too high, and in others the proportion of overweight and over-indulged is too high. Every country has a percentage of both categories. Bearing in mind the availability of supplies, either from local agricultural sources or from imports, a balanced diet for most communities can be achieved in theory. From a practical point of view, customs pertaining to food habit are strong and built in to the cultural pattern of the community. Nutritional education goes hand-in-hand with agricultural progress. The acceptance of new foods can often be extremely difficult. Many individuals know what is wrong with their diet, may know the correct balanced intake, but do not act on this knowledge.

As has been stated before, the expectant mother and her consort are often very keen to receive and absorb health facts for the well-being of their infant. So the terms mothercraft and parentcraft have been coined to cover this field of activity. Positive dental health is part of this programme. Dental caries is an epidemic disease, which is not hazardous to life. Therefore the community as a whole may not be very concerned, and even be apathetic, although an individual sufferer, especially with toothache, is much concerned. Family action is balanced diet, avoidance of sugar left on the teeth by sound oral hygiene, including regular brushing.

In those areas of the world where the fluoride content of the water is below one part per million, artificial adjustment to this standard level will have a beneficial effect on the state of the teeth in the community. This basic dental and medical recommendation to improve the state of children's teeth has not been universally welcomed, and in some instances there has been active hostile opposition. Here lies a paradoxical challenge to the health educator of the individual and the family wishing to prevent dental caries, yet faced with a community collectively reluctant to take the appropriate political action.

A drug is a chemical substance derived from natural or synthetic sources which has marked therapeutic effect in given doses. Drugs can be inhaled, ingested, injected, smoked, and applied direct. They can be tolerated in increasing doses. However, doses beyond the therapeutic level can lead to individual dependence on the drug.

Dependence can show itself in two forms; individuals are psychologically dependent on some drugs, and physically dependent on others. Withdrawal of drugs in the former case has no ill effect on the individual. Withdrawal of drugs in the latter can give rise to physical features of distress.

Certain drugs of dependence within cultural limits are socially acceptable. Tea and coffee are widely used as beverages, but some individuals can and do become very dependent on them, though with minimal clinical ill effects.

The drinking of alcoholic beverages, be they derived from the grape or the grain, within limits of quantity, is a social grace which lends a flair to culture. In certain personalities, especially under stress and in certain occupations, the intake of alcohol becomes an obsession, and the individual lives from one drink to the next. The social effect on occupation and family is disastrous. Many people have a drinking problem but not to the severe degree of being a chronic alcoholic, with its resultant hepatic cirrhosis and mental derangement. The incidence of those with drinking problems is not accurately known, but it is greater than many observers imagine.

A social pleasure often associated with the consumption of alcohol is smoking. The correlation between cigarette smoking and lung cancer is now well established. Chronic chest complaints and the habit of smoking are closely interlinked. Pipe and cigar smoking constitute health hazards but not to the same degree as cigarette smoking. In many parts of the world the smoking and chewing of hemp (*cannabis indicis*, hashish, marihuana) is part of the way of life.

In some countries possession of the drug is an offence against the law, the reasoning being that if an inadequate personality under stress in a drug-taking culture smokes hemp, then there is a grave risk that he or she will become dependent on other more sinister drugs. Others do not accept this postulation, and argue that the smoking of hemp in moderation is no greater hazard to health than the smoking of tobacco and the imbibing of alcohol.

Other drugs of dependence are the barbiturates, amphetamines, opium derivatives such as heroin, morphine and cocaine. If these drugs are taken habitually in ever increasing doses the individual can reach a state of total addiction with the resultant complete social degradation, and wreckage of the physical and mental state. The method of administration may be more important than the category of drug itself.

Thus the habits of cigarette smoking, drinking alcohol, and drug taking, if pushed to excess, are social diseases of great severity, and to be avoided. Health education, especially of the young, has an immense task in placing the health hazards of such activities fairly and squarely before all concerned. Society can take political action in keeping the production, distribution, and sale within strict legal boundaries. Some aspects need an international legal code. However, fundamentally the main body of world opinion must lay down the areas of acceptability unless there is to be complete degradation of mankind.

The excesses of affluence, such as overeating, lack of exercise, too much drinking and smoking, must be kept within moderate limits. A rigid attitude which prohibits these habits leads to excesses in subverse ways and defeats the object of control. A flexible, tolerant society can keep these habits within bounds.

Heart disease, especially coronary occlusive attacks in younger and middle-aged men in advanced societies, has its basic causation in these excesses of affluence. Again it must be stressed that the social effects of the sudden, early death of the breadwinner on the young family and the loss of educational investment for the community, are dire indeed. The health education techniques that can be built into the medical check situation for men is still in its early stages.

As the science of medicine develops, more sophisticated therapeutic methods and the epidemiology of the former killer diseases are better understood. Modern society with its technology brings to the fore the phenomenon of accidents. They can occur in the home, on the road, in industry, on the mountain, at sea, down the pothole, in the air—anywhere where mankind has his being, whatever his pursuit, whatever his activity. The severity of the injuries from an accident, important as they are to the individual, are not as important as the timing and the circumstances of the accident itself. The degree of fatigue, anger, depression, fear and other emotions in the individual, combined with the local environment at a given point in time, are the essential ingredients of an accident. Age plays its part. The inquisitive infant is at risk in the home to burning, poisoning, and falls; the adventuresome pre-school child to injury in the play area and on the road; the schoolchild and adult, in the same manner, to the transport accident and drowning. The young and middle-aged are liable to industrial accidents. The elderly are liable to falls in their homes. A comprehensive programme of education in human biology and the life sciences to children and young people is of paramount importance, with particular stress on adventure safety. Special attention to the training of teachers, architects and social workers in this field is essential. All members of the public should have a knowledge of the essentials of elementary first aid: the stoppage of bleeding, the commencement of resuscitation if breathing ceases, the immobilization of a fracture, the prevention of shock. All disciplines within a health service must be aware of and put into practice the principles of first aid.

The effect of extreme cold, in civilized countries, can have an adverse effect, especially on the very young and the old. A sudden nocturnal fall in room temperature leads to a lowering of the body temperature below 35°C (95°F)—the resultant condition being known as accidental hypothermia. Preventive action lies with health and social workers to anticipate this possible social tragedy by taking appropriate action to boost heating arrangements within the house, particularly in bedrooms. Advice to the mothers of young infants and to old people in the autumn and early winter to initiate action is of paramount importance, such as the prudent use of supplementary kits of mobile heating units, sleeping bags, blankets.

The techniques of health education are varied and are still evolving.

1. Eyeball to eyeball situation. Whenever a member of the health disciplines, medical practitioner, nurse, health officer,

E

ambulance attendant or home help, is face-to-face with a patient, then informal health advice may be given. These circumstances have the optimum impact.

2. Group discussion and demonstrations with visual aids present the subject and allow a two-way exchange of views on an informal basis between all participants.

3. The set lecture to a large audience can be dull and have minimal effect. The amount of knowledge ingested is inversely proportional to the size of the gathering. However, with the judicious and flexible use of visual aids, such as films, and breaking the lecture into shorter talks with two or more speakers, a fruitful panel session can evolve.

4. Pamphlets. In the middle of the nineteenth century in north-west England, when enlightened members of the community became concerned about infant ill health, pamphlets on child care were distributed. The result was a failure. It was then decided to have a visitor call on mothers with young children to give advice on health matters; thus the profession of health visiting was born. This experience with pamphlets on health information is still true well over a hundred years later. Posters, either on one theme or varied to give the viewer a choice, can be used in the surgery, clinic or public place.

5. Articles. The well written article in newspapers and magazines, especially those catering for female interests, has a part to play in a progressive health education programme. The correspondence column, if handled intelligently, provides a strong back-up to previous health articles.

6. Health Exhibitions. Such an enterprise is costly in time, money, and personnel if it is to be produced and staged to a high standard. The promoters must be prepared for this outlay, otherwise it is not worth the effort.

7. Mass Media. The radio and television media have a high degree of influence for good throughout the world. Their approach can be either direct with documentary programmes on given health subjects, or correct health advice and techniques can be introduced indirectly into other programmes, including the drama situation.

Closed circuit television is being explored in its role in health education. Its future has immense possibilities.

In advanced societies the priorities for a health education programme are as follows:

Smoking	Sex Education	Personal Hygiene
Alcoholism	Venereal Disease	Tooth Decay
Drugs	Birth Control	Accident Prevention

The community physician must always be studying mortality and morbidity data in order to discern trends of social disease in order that the emphasis and direction of the health education programme can be evaluated so as to achieve maximum return on investment of time and resources.

REFERENCES

Gardiner, A. W., Roylance, P. J. (1970) *New Safety and First Aid*. Pan Books, London.

H.M.S.O. (1968) *A Handbook of Health Education*.

Miles, S., Roylance, P. J. (1970) *Teaching First Aid*. Bailliere, Tindall and Cassell.

7

The Interface between Health and Social Services

THE discipline of medicine is intertwined with society and the services organized by that society in given communities. Some prescriptions for social therapy are dispensed by teams under medical direction, while others are dispensed by teams under non-medical direction but, it is hoped, with medical advice. Academic debate surrounds the argument where the dividing line between these teams should be. In practice the essential aim and object of any health service is the welfare of the patient. The postulation of socio-medical situations and their solutions has necessitated reference to personal health and social welfare services.

The length of time that the majority of patients spend in hospital is comparatively short. Yet the resources both in personnel and money spent in the hospital field attracts dramatic attention. The hospital serves its community or catchment area by investigating, establishing the diagnosis, and treating patients both on an out-patient and in-patient basis. In the advanced societies, medicine has tended to follow a scientific and technological bias, which seems to be concentrated in the hospital service. In the developing communities, the sociological role of the hospital is still very much to the fore. In any community there must be balance between the sociological and scientific approach in providing a comprehensive health service.

In Great Britain the foundations of the health service rest firmly on the family doctor, who is the personal physician to an individual and his family. Some argue that the physician of first contact is a generalist, not a specialist in medicine, and hence the descriptive term—general practitioner. Others argue that the art, science, and vocational calling of general practice, that is medical practice in the community, is a speciality in its own right. The medical ethic in the United Kingdom holds the premise that no specialist or consultant can see a patient by direct contact, but must be so referred by a family doctor. There are a few agreed exceptions to

52

this ethical code. If a social worker in contact with a client feels that a specialist opinion must be obtained, the correct approach is by way of the family doctor who, if he is agreeable, will make the necessary arrangements. Family doctors work together in partnerships either in a group practice or health centre. A minority have clinical appointments within the hospitals.

A health centre is a community-orientated health establishment where the practitioners of primary medical care function. A health centre in England and Wales is the responsibility of the local community; in Scotland it is the responsibility of the central government. A group practice is established and administered by a partnership of family doctors. Functionally there are few differences. The family doctor is the leader of a community sociomedical team. Nurses in the community may work entirely with one partnership and care for only patients of that practice. This arrangement is known as attachment and is dependent on the ecology of the area. Partial attachment or liaison arrangements exist where the community nurses see patients of other practices. Both sets of arrangements have two limiting factors, firstly the availability of nursing staff and secondly the personalities involved. These schemes are evolutionary in character at the present time and may never be complete, the reasoning being that individuals move from one community to another in a modern society and therefore may not always have a personal physician. The community nurses will be in contact with them and be working through particular episodes, before the family has formed a professional relationship with a personal medical attendant. The work relationship between the family doctor and the community nurse can take two forms:

1. Delegation. The patient consults the physician of first contact, who outlines the policy of therapy, and the community nurse implements.
2. Selection. The patient calls at the practice premises and, not necessarily on the primary visit, is seen by a member of the nursing team, who decides on the evidence whether the patient should be seen by the primary care physician or not. It may well be that the community nurse of the future will visit a patient in his own home and report her findings to the primary care physician, so that appropriate therapy can be initiated. There are ethical considerations in this

procedure pertaining to the clinical responsibility of the medical practitioner.

The composition of the community team in support of the primary care physician is as follows:

1. Surgery Nurse or Clinical Nurse Attendant, who may co-ordinate the clinical arrangements within the group practice or health centre. A degree of seniority rests on this individual with related responsibilities. Some general practitioners and community physicians take the view that a lay administrative practice manager may be the appropriate officer for the future.

2. Health Visitor. A health visitor is a social worker with a predominantly nursing background. She is the most important all-purpose health worker whose main role is that of family adviser and immediate co-ordinator of social welfare services.

3. Home Nurse or District Nurse. The basic nursing qualifications with additional tuition for district nursing is the requirement. Both men and women form this group and their role is primarily administering therapy and general nursing care in the home. Limited social welfare action is also undertaken. These nurses must be supported by the provision of appropriate nursing equipment. Night nursing schemes can be established for seriously ill patients prior to admission to hospital.

4. Domiciliary Midwife. A trained midwife is nearly always a trained nurse as well. She may also be trained in district nursing procedures. In Great Britain at the time of writing, with the increase in the proportion of hospital confinements, integrated obstetric nursing training and comprehensive maternity schemes are being evolved, so that the care of the mother and newly born infant is as complete as possible.

5. Nursing Auxiliary. These are individuals who have undertaken a modified course of training in practical nursing care.

6. Nursing Ancillary. Bath attendants and other individuals with nursing experience, who can assist the district nurses.

7. Home Help. It is considered by many, even in authority, that a home help is a social worker. In practice a home help

is required to give loving care and attention to patients and act as a substitute for relatives. She can keep a home running during acute and chronic illness and in the puerperium.

(a) Good Neighbour. If a home help is not available, and an elderly person needs help with shopping, lighting of fires, making of beds, etc., a good neighbour can be retained to carry out these tasks for a fee.

(b) Night Sitter. If a sick person is being nursed and cared for in his own home and (i) is awaiting urgent admission to hospital and no bed is available immediately, then in the absence of relatives a nocturnal home help or night sitter is indicated; (ii) has a chronic terminal illness and is being cared for devotedly by relatives, the latter after several nights without sleep become very exhausted. A night sitter would give them one or two nights' respite.

The health visiting profession came into being to advise mothers about the care of their infants. A parallel development historically was the provision of milk depots for these infants. From these foundations, maternity and child health clinics have been established. At these sessions a team of doctors with special experience in child health, including knowledge of developmental medicine, and health visitors examine, counsel, and advise mothers about child care. Special attention is given to feeding, screening procedures, and the implementation of immunization protection programmes. It has been argued that the family doctor can undertake this role. This postulation is accepted, but those who wish to practise child health techniques must undertake appropriate postgraduate training and have the necessary time to give to this work. In the same building supplies of dried milk and vitamin supplements can be made available, but their distribution should not be the function of the child health clinic staff.

The expectant mother can receive her antenatal care at either antenatal sessions with mothercraft classes at these clinics, or by way of special out-patient facilities provided at a maternity unit. The primary medical care physician with a community midwife is in a position to practise this antenatel care. Expectant mothers are a priority group for dental care and treatment. Special social welfare arrangements are needed for the homeless, unsupported mother. The day care of the child for an unsupported mother can be arranged with a child minder, day nursery or crèche. Whatever method is provided, medical and nursing surveillance is necessary for both staff and children concerned.

A special transport or ambulance service for the conveyance of sick and injured persons is an integral part of any health service. It has two main tasks, firstly to convey sick persons from their homes to hospital and back, secondly to render professional first aid and remove injured casualties from the site of an episode to a major accident centre. An ambulance service can use multi-purpose vehicles to meet both requirements. However, geography and the degree of urbanization may determine separately designed and equipped transport for each role. The requirements as to the training of ambulance driver/attendants, including resuscitative techniques, are the subject of active review and improvement. Communication by fixed telephone lines, teleprinters, and radio telephones, is an essential component of a modern ambulance service.

Sick persons in their own homes have need of additional supportive services:

1. Recuperative holiday or convalescence after an illness is very necessary in spite of the advances of scientific medicine. Periods of fourteen to twenty-eight days in an appropriate home recommended on medical advice aid and promote recovery.

2. Chiropody. If an individual is crippled by a foot disorder, then social imprisonment and isolation in his own home can result. A domiciliary visit and treatment by a qualified chiropodist is sound preventive action, and subsequent visits for chiropodial treatment at a clinic or surgery may follow. Priority categories for such treatment are schoolchildren, expectant mothers, the chronically physically handicapped, the elderly, and sufferers from specific medical conditions, e.g. *diabetes mellitus*.

The term mentally disordered includes the mentally ill, subnormal and severely subnormal and the psychopathic personality. The mentally disordered have always been in society. Mental hospitals or asylums are comparatively recent establishments with maximum development during the last two hundred years. Many societies in the world retain and support their mentally sick and afflicted within their own families and communities. Some patients with acute mental illnesses need in-patient hospital care and intensive treatment. Others may not require to be admitted, and here day hospital attendance and therapy, for patients living in their own homes, can be beneficial. If a mentally ill patient cannot return to his own home then residential accommodation in a hostel is required. He can then either be boarded out in another person's home or cared for in a sheltered flatlet. He may be fit to follow an occupation while living in sheltered and supportive surroundings. Day centres and sheltered workshops without intensive medical therapy can provide craft and occupational pursuits. Mental health social work teams under psychiatric direction can undertake deep and supportive case work with mentally ill patients.

The mentally subnormal can be trained from the early age of two to three years. Pre-nursery units within special schools can provide a high degree of social teaching. Educative and social pursuits can be continued up to the age of sixteen. Special care units for severely physically handicapped and hyperactive subnormals are attached to modern special schools. Adult training centres provide simple work situations and continued social and educational activities for leavers from both the subnormal and educational subnormal special schools. Mental health social workers again have a role in counselling and supporting the families with a subnormal individual. Medical surveillance and assessment is an essential requirement because of the high incidence of associated handicapping conditions. Residential care by either weekly boarding units, hostels, or fostering arrangements may be required for subnormals of all ages if the social conditions in their own homes are inadequate. Permanent hospital placement is only necessary if continued nursing care is prescribed. It is to be appreciated that this latter provision is an integral part of a comprehensive mental health programme.

As previously mentioned, a school psychological service will detect those children who have learning difficulties. However, some of these children are so disturbed that psychiatric diagnosis and psychotherapy are indicated as an essential part of a child psychiatric service. Historically these two services merge and can operate as a family advice establishment, known as the child guidance service. The component staff traditionally are a child psychiatrist, educational psychologist and psychiatric social workers. The service can be based either in the community or at a hospital. The former has advantages in that it is closely linked with the child health clinics and schools; the latter has the benefit of access to hospital beds.

There is no true division between health and social services, since an individual in need of help cannot determine what service he or she needs. There must be a mutually respected partnership, so that a team approach of different skills and disciplines is achieved.

REFERENCES

H.M.S.O. (1969) *Nursing Attachments to General Practice.*

The Dan Mason Nursing Research Committee (1970) *Home from Hospital.*

Warren, M. D. (1970) A Synoptic History of Health and Related Services 1801–1969. *The Medical Officer,* **17,** 229–232.

Part Two   Public Health

8

Environmental Public Health

INDIVIDUAL man, as the community in which he lives, requires a pure water supply, clean food and reliable sewage and refuse disposal. If the methods and systems are not adequate then men will foul the soil, rivers, sea and air by which he lives. This fouling, by axiom, is a hazard to the health of both the individual and the community. The ideal *milieu* for disease. It follows that environmental health and sanitary measures are the most fundamental of all community health services.

The conservation of the world's natural resources is an international responsibility. The preservation involved and the disposal of waste is not the prerogative of medical men, though they have a part to play. The practitioners of the disciplines of the pure sciences of physics, chemistry, biology and geology, and of the applied sciences and technologies, including architecture, engineering and their planning sub-disciplines, should all be actively concerned and involved. Public health, engineering and food technology are in the forefront of this movement.

Sanitary measures are often implemented by local communities within the structure of legalization enacted by society as a whole. Local communities either themselves organize or create a local authority to provide, maintain and service these sanitary measures.

These authorities should provide the necessary public sewers to drain their district properly and to deal with sewage either at a sewage disposal works or elsewhere. They may require any sewer to be so constructed that it forms part of a general sewage system. A public sewer can be closed or altered to meet changes in needs, but equally effective alternatives must be made available. These sewers must be cleansed and emptied. Powers may be taken to recover costs for their upkeep. Facilities must be afforded to factories to drain effluents into public sewers as long as it is not harmful to health nor would cause other damage. Injurious matter must not be passed into the sewers so as to cause damage to, or hold back, the contents, nor should any variety of petroleum spirit or calcium carbide be introduced.

61

The community should be able to hold land for the purpose of treating sewage: they may dispose of fouled water after purification into streams, canals, ponds or lakes. New buildings must be provided with drains. Buildings can be required to have adequate closet accommodation. If these are insufficient or are in need of repair or replacement, the owner can be compelled to remedy the situation.

Every factory should be supplied with sufficient and satisfactory sanitary accommodation for persons of each sex, if this should be necessary. All drains, sewers, cesspools and sanitary conveniences have to be maintained in such a condition that they are not prejudicial to health or creating a nuisance. Special attention to design, position, and access for physically handicapped persons should be observed. Dangerous or dilapidated buildings must be either repaired or demolished.

Public buildings are required to have adequate exits, entrances, passages and gangways to give satisfactory ingress and egress for the safety of the public; all such means must be kept free and unobstructed with special provision for the physically handicapped. Such buildings are theatres, halls, restaurants, shops, stores, warehouses, clubs, schools, and places of public worship. There must be adequate means of escape in case of fire in any building which exceeds two storeys in height and in which the floor of any upper storey is more than twenty feet above the ground, and which is let in flats or tenements, or used as an inn, hotel, boarding house, hospital, nursing home, day or boarding school, children's home or similar establishment; or if it is used as a restaurant, shop, store, or warehouse, and has on any upper floor sleeping accommodation for persons employed on the premises.

Removal of house refuse and cleansing of earth closets, privies, ashpits or cesspools, has to be arranged. Trade refuse can also be dealt with, but a charge may or may not be made. Owners or occupiers of premises can be required to provide dustbins. Refuse receptacles should be provided in the streets.

Arrangements may be made for the tipping of refuse or the provision of refuse destruction apparatus. The practice of totting or sorting over refuse for gain is to be discouraged.

Streets should be swept and washed regularly. Common passages and courts which are not a highway should be kept clear and free of rubbish. Accumulations of noxious matter and the manure should be removed periodically from stables. Such nuisances as slush, filth, dust and ashes, can be controlled and eliminated. The keeping of animals can be held to standards that are not prejudicial to health. The removal or conveyance through the streets of any faecal, noxious or offensive matter must be controlled, and the receptacle or vehicle must be of sound construction to prevent the escape of liquid: if the liquid does escape it can be required to be cleaned up.

Premises which are in such a filthy or unwholesome condition as to be prejudicial to health, or are verminous, can be cleaned up by notice on the owner or occupier, or in default by community services who can recover the cost. Filthy and verminous articles can be dealt with in the same way. Cleansing stations can be set up where verminous persons and their clothing can be cleaned free of charge. Public sanitary conveniences may be provided by the community, who may require the owners and occupiers of any inn, public or refreshment house, or place of public entertainment, to provide a reasonable number of sanitary conveniences. Again special arrangements should be made for the physically handicapped.

Nuisances

The community can arrange for its geographical area to be inspected for the detection of nuisances, which can be defined as:

1. Any premises in such a state as to be prejudicial to health or a nuisance.
2. Any animal so kept in such a place or like manner.
3. Any deleterious accumulation or deposit.
4. Any dust or effluvia caused by any trade, business, manufacture or process, and being prejudicial to the health or a nuisance to the inhabitants of the neighbourhood.
5. Any workplace which is not provided with sufficient means of ventilation or in which sufficient ventilation is not maintained, or which is not kept clean or not kept free from noxious effluvia, or which is overcrowded while work is carried on.

Other nuisances can include insanitary cisterns, ditches, ponds and watercourses, as well as tents, vans and sheds.

The community takes legal steps to abate nuisances on the person causing the nuisance or the owner or occupier of the premises. In structural nuisances the notice must be served on the owner.

Smoke Nuisances

Smoke nuisances arise where smoke, soot, ash or grit are emitted from the chimneys of boilers or industrial plant in such quantities that they cause a nuisance to local inhabitants. Above certain defined shades of darkness, smoke from dwelling-houses, as well as from industrial plants can be dealt with as a nuisance.

On detection an abatement notice is served as for any other statutory nuisance and similar court action follows if it is not complied with and provided the defendant does not show that all practicable steps have been taken to prevent the nuisance.

Smoke control areas achieve considerable improvement in that all premises must use only smokeless fuels and other non-smoking sources of energy. These measures apply to both domestic premises and industrial concerns.

Noise Nuisance

Some noise must be accepted as within tolerable limits to normal individuals, otherwise life would not be able to go on. The movement of traffic, the shutting of doors, the rattling of bottles, all are commonplace. However, excess noise can be a nuisance and unreasonable: the juke box from the local café, high spirits and shouting from the dance hall, frequent aircraft over cities at night. Society has yet to come to terms with nosie. For the anxious and the depressed, noise can be an adverse nuisance to their health.

Offensive trades

The community may make strict regulations about the following trades: Blood-boiler, blood-drier, bone-boiler, fat-extractor, fat-melter, fell-monger, glue-maker, gut-scraper, rag-and-bone-dealer, size-maker, soap-boiler, tallow-melter, tripe-boiler. Fish frying can also be limited.

REFERENCES

The Standing Medical Advisory Committee for the Central Health Services Council and the Minister of Health (1968) *Communicable Diseases Contracted outside Great Britain.*

Wilcocks, C. (1970) *Imported Tropical Diseases Health Trends*, 2, 91.

9

Prevention and Control of Infectious Disease

EPIDEMIOLOGY has been defined as the study of the natural history of infectious disease. It would be more appropriate to replace the word 'infectious' by 'community', as there are a variety of medical conditions which are caused by, or linked with, a specific way of communal life. Most attention up to now has been paid to infection, but epidemiological principles applied to non-infectious entities such as cancer, coronary disease, congenital defects, diabetes and mental illness, have been of considerable scientific and practical importance. Epidemics vary in severity and extent. An epidemic starts when the governing factors coincide in being at their optimum. The factors can be likened to the seed, the soil and the climate. There is an increase in the power of the causal organisms to infect; a decrease in resistance or an increase in susceptibility of the population at risk, and lastly some change in the climate or environment, such as an increase in humidity or the massing or assembling of a large number of persons who are open to infection.

The epidemic slows or stops when the reverse occurs of the factors which favour spread. This halt occurs naturally or as a result of human intervention. The factors pertaining to cessation are the dispersal of the groups at risk, a reduction in the community susceptibility, possibly aided by artificial measures, the exhaustion of the supply of susceptibles and a decrease in the effectiveness of the causal organisms.

Artificial intervention can be by the vaccination and isolation of contacts as in an outbreak of smallpox; by immunization, by boiling or disinfecting a water supply in the face of epidemic typhoid or cholera or, in an episode of food poisoning, by controlling and modifying procedures in the manufacture or distribution of food.

The spread of infection derives from the presence of a source of infection, the routes of infection and the availability of susceptible recipients. Control depends upon accurate and rapid diagnosis, so

F

that the cause is recognized. Where appropriate this is followed by vigorous and efficient tracing of contacts who are brought under surveillance and control. The source of infection exists somewhere: it will remain a risk and will be liable to cause trouble again until it is identified and neutralized. The routes of infection must be discovered and all who lie in the path must be considered potentially at risk until control is established.

If infectious disease is to be controlled the work has to be done properly. Half-done work is ineffective and therefore useless. If the measures instituted are seen to be ineffective there is a problem of loss of confidence among the community with all its consequences, including the risk of loss of public collaboration with the community's health adviser, possibly under worsening conditions.

For all practical purposes there is no infectious disease which can be controlled without some participation by the community at risk. The powers given to any health administration do not, and cannot, permit total control under penal conditions. The reasons, which on reflection are obvious, are firstly that the law is usually not up-to-date in the specific measures it sets out for infectious disease control and secondly that it would be necessary to provide an enormous staff for constant surveillance, particularly of those anti-social families in homes where fecklessness and ignorance reinforce the onslaught of infection, especially on ill-cared-for children.

Participation and collaboration are secured by health education designed to create a well-informed community attuned to receiving advice on health matters. Fear of infectious disease is still prevalent. It is reduced or abolished by explanation of the situation to the man in the street in language which he understands.

The introduction of control measures must be accompanied by a clear and simple explanation of the reasons. The controls themselves must also be simple and clearly understood and be firmly applied. It is always possible to relax conditions at a later date, but it is almost impossible to apply gradually increasing and more restrictive control.

In dealing with the source of infection, contact routes must be interrupted and the infected individual isolated forthwith. Those in attendance on him in isolation must not be susceptible and so should be either naturally immune or fully immunized. If the patient is isolated at home it is necessary to give detailed instructions to the relatives and attendants on action to prevent the spread of disease. The situation is more complex in dealing with healthy carriers of such diseases as dysentery or salmonellosis. These carriers may need most careful explanations before they can understand the real reason why their movements or actions have to be restricted at a time when they feel perfectly well. Quite obviously such carriers of bowel-borne disease, if they have access to water-borne sanitation, need little restriction other than instruction in correct hand hygiene after defaecation. Even food-handling can be permitted provided that the individual is of a sufficient level of intelligence and reliability.

Different diseases demand different procedures. The control of infectious disease may be attempted by mass measures of simple type applied to all and sundry. Such action as dispersal of schools, the closing of cinemas and swimming baths, and mass prohibitions of one sort or another are rarely effective because they are often by-passed. Their main result is to disrupt the ordinary life of the community and so cloud the background scene before which the infectious disease episode is being played. The alternative is to study the natural history of the outbreak, to make an intelligent appreciation of the situation and then to apply selective action designed to achieve its effect with the minimum of interruption of the normal way of life. This alternative method means much harder work, more considered judgement and a sound existing standard of health education in the community so that the people will accept the advice of their community physician, and particularly his reassurance and confidence in the absence of more heroic measures such as they may have experienced elsewhere in the past.

Notification of certain infectious diseases is a legal requirement in Great Britain. However, personal and hospital physicians may not always notify the community physician and a degree of under-notification for certain diseases could well exist. The incidence of pathogenic identifications in the microbiological service will give a firm lead on infections in a community. On this information appropriate action can be considered in order to achieve control and prevent further spread. Certain infectious diseases are endemic and are relatively harmless if they are properly treated and the side effects avoided. Communities become acclimatized to certain infectious diseases and by the acquisition of so-called herd immunity suffer less than new populations who have never been exposed to infection.

In Europe the population is acclimatized to a group of diseases which nowadays are relatively harmless. These include rubella, chickenpox and mumps. No measures of control are necessary as it is accepted that the risk is so widespread and the results so insignificant that it is better for all to acquire natural immunity by infection. Certain *sequelae* of rubella in pregnant women make it even more desirable that all girls should either acquire natural immunity or be so protected by immunization before exposure to pregnancy. Some other diseases, notably measles and whooping-cough, are endemic and can become serious by reason of their complications. Measures to control them would be widespread and cumbersome. Modern therapy is effective with the complications in most instances. However, immunization programmes against both diseases give partial control in that milder clinical features follow.

In principle, the control of all infectious disease is by the identification of those individuals incubating the condition, the clinical cases and also the carriers, and then the isolation of these individuals so that they are unable to infect others. It is a helpful refinement to give protective immunization either generally or to particular groups at risk. Isolation as a measure of control is relative.

Smallpox in its more severe form is a killing disease. As a result of its grave consequences the strictest quarantine is justifiable, together with a vigorous policy of the vaccination of all contacts, potential or actual. Chickenpox is little more than a social nuisance and isolation of cases until the last scab has fallen off is sufficient action without any contact-tracing. The one point which is really significant to remember is that chickenpox and smallpox are different diagnoses of pock disease, even though the latter may be infrequent in a particular country.

Infectious Disease

That the major infections have been largely eliminated in some parts of the world does not mean that we can ignore their significance. Epidemic infection is always a menace, sometimes overwhelming, sometimes lurking to strike. The menace remains in the world, but medical and scientific advances allow preventive measures to be successfully introduced.

The effect on primitive populations living only at subsistence levels is quite different from the effect on civilized communities who live in a scientifically controlled environment with adequate economic, medical and social resources.

The evolution of a community from being agrarian orientated to becoming industrially based involves an epidemiological component.

If a community traditionally living on the borderline of hunger is freed from the threat of epidemic disease, the death-rate falls, there are more survivors, the fertility of those hitherto debilitated increases and the size of the population goes up by the survival of adults and infants who would otherwise have died, in addition to the increased number of births of children who have a better chance of growing up. The simple mathematics are that there are and will be extra mouths to feed in a community which previously was limited by hunger.

The greater energy given to the survivors will permit a better agricultural output, but even with interim agricultural training and assistance these steps will not provide enough food for the increased population. Under these circumstances the only answer is emigration, that is disruption of the community. Often it is the young, energetic and adventuresome who emigrate.

Food may be imported from abroad, which can be purchased only by increasing exports. The export of saleable raw materials or of valuable manufactures is encouraged. The development of such exports creates the urgent need for extra hands in factories, in mines and quarries yielding export minerals, on plantations and in other agricultural fields. Adequate housing and other social needs for the workpeople cannot be met for years. Slum or shanty conditions are created, with consequent new opportunities for community disease. The wheel turns full circle and urban infectious disease begins to take its toll in mortality and morbidity. There is a collapse of personal standards under the pressure of a squalid environment. Tuberculosis, bowel-borne and fly-carried infection and venereal disease flourish amid a way of life beset by medico-social problems. If ethnic groups move from their country of origin to another country, these circumstances can arise if the numbers involved are not controlled so as to allow harmonious adaptation and assimilation in the host group.

Food-borne disease

The present supply of food to urban populations is so complex that it is remarkable not that there is so much breakdown in the system, but so little. This is the result of a combination of

70 PUBLIC AND COMMUNITY HEALTH

legislation on conduct and standards, health education and raised personal standards. Though much has been done, much has yet to be done in advancing the training and education of all who have to do with food.

Food-borne disease may be due to infected ingredients in the food or to mishandling or unhygienic conduct leading to the introduction of infection from outside. Undoubtedly it is the human factor which presents most difficulty in food poisoning. For the social problem is a combined one involving health education, the level of intelligence of the food-handlers, the quality of management, industrial discipline and all that goes with it, and the stimulus or otherwise of the working environment.

In this connexion it is beyond all doubt that trained staff constantly practising hygiene measures are far safer than the untrained, who rely on what they remember, and much that they have half forgotten, of what they were taught when working with mother at home or in the domestic science class at school.

It is useless to expect food-handlers to maintain hygiene standards if facilities are defective or do not exist. To do its job a wash basin must be well maintained and sited immediately outside a water closet, so that those who are about to leave are prompted to wash by its immediate presence. The basin must be clean, there must be hot and cold water, soap, nail brush and clean towels, or the equivalent in paper towels or hand dryers. The staff must be told of the health hazards which exist. They should notify all ill health, particularly diarrhoea and septic conditions such as boils and infected skin lesions due to streptococci or staphylococci.

The purpose behind all kitchen processes should be clearly explained, if not already known. The principles underlying refrigeration, the avoidance of reheating of food, the consequences of breakdown in personal hygiene, the reasons for certain steps in washing dishes and utensils, the risks from dust, pests and vermin, once properly taught and understood mean an easier and improved standard of food processes. The alternative is trouble which, if serious enough, makes newspaper headlines, destroys confidence and can lead to litigation.

Food poisoning is due to direct bacteriological action, to bacteriological exotoxins, or occasionally to chemical agents. The picture is one of simultaneous cases with linked onset in which investigation reveals one significant common factor.

The human carrier is the commonest cause of the outbreak,

even if evidence is available that the prime product may have been infected, for example the live animal prior to slaughter. Bowel-borne salmonellosis or staphylococcal exotoxin from skin or nasal conditions and toxins from *Clostridium welchii* spores are the most frequent causes of episodes. All are due to some breach in hygienic conduct. Rats and mice can act as carriers of salmonellosis and infect food with their droppings. Duck eggs can be contaminated in the oviduct. Flies with fouled legs and bodies become a risk when they have had previous access to such reservoirs of infection as privies and middens.

Foodstuffs such as meat, milk products and egg albumen, are but another variant of the nutrient culture media used for growing bacteria in the laboratory: with suitable conditions of temperature and moisture they too will rapidly grow any inoculum of pathogenic bacteria.

Shellfish are sometimes incriminated in food poisoning out-breaks. They can cause trouble by acting as the medium for growing introduced pathogenic bacteria in the same way that mishandling will infest other food. They also have certain inherent toxins, usually in the gonads at certain seasons: these toxins can cause poisoning, usually with the complication of utricaria and sometimes with neurotrophic symptoms. The third hazard is that if shellfish are gathered in areas polluted by sewage there is a risk that they may contain pathogenic bacteria. Such gathering must be pro-hibited and no sympathy should be wasted on complainants who have breached the law made for their specific protection. Shellfish can be cleansed after being gathered from approved clean layings.

Botulism is an extremely rare and fatal form of food poisoning. It is due to the exotoxin of *B. botulinus*. The toxin is a neurotrophic poison of the motor nervous system which is fatal in a week. The risk is associated with the preparation of *Sauerkraut* and the manufacture of some varieties of continental sausage.

Enteric Fever

Typhoid and paratyphoid fever are diseases spread by the con-tamination of water or milk by *S. typhi* and *S. paratyphi* A and B. The disease is bowel-borne. No drug is specific though chloram-phenicol abates the symptoms. The bacterium can be demon-strated in the bowel after a course of treatment has ceased. Carriers tend to be chronic either as bowel or urinary excretors.

Personal hygiene, efficient disposal of excreta and fly control are essential to eliminate the risk of spread. In practice it is undesirable to employ carriers on waterworks, in dairies and as food handlers. All known carriers should be kept under surveillance at intervals to determine if and when they cease to excrete. The disease is still present in many countries, thus travellers and holiday-makers are at special risk. Prophylaxis is general in the provision of safe water, safe milk, and proper food hygiene. Personal protection can be given and repeated by injections with TAB vaccine, which combines antigens for typhoid and for paratyphoid A and B.

Nasopharyngeal infections

The common cold is a minor, but widespread, virus infection, which constitutes a sizeable proportion of all illness. The common cold is uncontrollable. The incubation period is short. Complete recovery occurs in a few days. The social significance is the enormous brief morbidity with consequent economic loss. It would not be possible to ask all potential cases to remain at home in isolation, as the resulting disruption of activity would be as great as, or greater than, that caused by the illness itself. The common cold is but one of a wide spectrum of coryza viruses, including the influenza group. Influenza has been known for centuries. There are many strains of influenza of which most are relatively harmless. At intervals a particularly virulent strain appears and causes an epidemic, or even one which spreads throughout the world to cause a pandemic. The greatest pandemic occurred in 1918–19 when there were twenty million deaths; more people lost their lives than were killed in the whole of the previous four years of the Great War. Influenza can be directly fatal or can be synergistic to raise the death rate. Pandemics of benign types can be traced from Asia and Australia to America and Europe. From this it was possible to predict that the condition would run a harmless course. In general this is so, but there are disproportionate numbers of deaths of old people due to bronchitis and pneumonia.

It is prudent that sufferers from chest and heart complaints should receive personal protection during the autumn months. In addition essential health, transport, and emergency service personnel should be offered such protection.

Diphtheria is almost extinct in the advanced countries due to the introduction of general immunization over the last three to four decades. The few cases and even smaller number of deaths occur among the unimmunized. Protection is almost entirely effective, but the picture remains satisfactory only while the great majority of children continue to be immunized.

Without immunization, the disease can be rapidly fatal even though antitoxin can be given. To be fully effective antitoxin must be given in adequate doses, after prior testing for sensitivity, as soon as the disease is suspected. Delay or under-dosing, until the bacteriological diagnosis is complete may lead to a fatality or complications which could have been avoided. Besides the risk of death there is that of disability by muscular paralysis affecting the heart, the eye, the soft palate and other areas of the body. Control means interruption of school and community life until the contacts have been traced and placed under surveillance. It should be noted that immunization against diphtheria is immunization against the toxin and not against the organism itself.

Measles for several decades has been considered to be the most menacing of the common infectious diseases. This is due to the complications rather than to the main complaint: these include respiratory infection, notably broncho-pneumonia, middle ear and eye infection, and post-infective encephalitis. The sulphonamides and the antibiotics have altered the picture. The advent of immunization programmes against measles is continuing this progress. In past years measles, when introduced to new populations which had no resistance, killed many of those infected.

Rubella, German measles, was formerly considered to be merely a minor complaint little different from a common cold with a rash. Observation in Australia three decades ago showed the relationship of German measles in the expectant mother in the first trimester of pregnancy to the occurrence of defects and deformities in the developing foetus. Under these circumstances the disease at once assumed a new significance. If the mother is a contact, then her antibody *titre* to rubella determines further action as to whether she should be protected with gamma globulin, or whether there are strong medical grounds for the termination of the pregnancy. This situation produces stress and anxiety and needs firm, sympathetic advice by the professional attendants. If a severely damaged child is born then the complete range of medico-social services necessary for its care will be required, with consequent involvement of staff, finance and facilities which could have been avoided, and effort given to help others if only control of such infection can be achieved. There is a strong hope that with the advent of an attenuated live rubella vaccine young women may be protected. The criteria of timing as to whether such a procedure is a school leaving or wedding present has yet to be defined.

Plague is transmitted by rat fleas. A mortality of rats precedes the first human cases by a fortnight. The fleas leave the dying rats to feed on and so infect other rats or human beings. In the pneumonic variety of plague the infection is transmitted direct by droplet infection. Control consists of surveying the rat-flea population ratio for a possible increase in the plague flea *Xenopsylla cheopsis* and a constant endeavour to eliminate rats.

When the disease occurs there must be isolation of patients and contacts.

Plague is recorded throughout history. A third of the population of Britain died in the Black Death of 1348 so that the whole population and social structure of the country was altered. The Great Plague of London in 1665 was the last great manifestation of the disease in Britain.

Plague remains a potential menace particularly when rats flourish under conditions of gross population disturbance, famine and the disruption of hygienic measures among civilian communities exposed to war.

Smallpox in Europe has now become an insignificant and exotic importation whose social significance lies only in the disruption of community life caused by the necessary control measures and by the unreasoning demands of the general population for immediate vaccination when they realize, too late, the significance of their own former apathetic attitude to protection by vaccination and re-vaccination.

Typhus is transmitted by the louse. Louse-borne typhus has been the scourge of armies in the field, of refugees herded together in confusion and of all those who live huddled together in squalor. Its social significance is that the louse exists everywhere and that the disease is very often fatal, more particularly in the debilitated. The introduction of the disease is followed by rapid spread. Control is achieved by constant attack to reduce the louse population and of intensive delousing campaigns in any community emergency such as an earthquake or other national disaster.

Huge epidemics have been recorded of which that in Ireland in the 1840s and in the Balkans in the 1914–18 War are the best known.

Typhus was formerly the common inhabitant of our prisons.

Outbreaks of 'Jail Fever' during trials in the eighteenth century carried off prisoners, lawyers, judges and spectators with impartial efficiency. While that is past history, the present demand for elaborate feminine hair styles favours the growth of the head louse so that the vector remains active in the community.

Malaria is a preventable disease which kills millions of people each year and by the morbidity among countless others causes widespread economic and social distress and inefficiency throughout many tropical and sub-tropical countries. Personal physicians in temperate climes far from malarious areas should always be alert to the disease, especially in recently returned air travellers.

The enormous death rate includes many infants so that the continuity of the population itself may be threatened and not able to replace itself as fertility is decreased. The survivors suffer from chronic anaemia to a varying degree. In consequence they are less fit for the daily task and less able to resist disease. Prevention by prophylactic drugs and by the elimination of the anopheles mosquito brings a changed social problem. Whereas in the past the population has been able to adjust itself to the limits of its environment, with the introduction of modern preventive measures it increases in size disproportionately both by the survival of those who would previously have died and by the fertility of those no longer disabled by chronic malaria.

Cholera is an infectious water-borne bowel infection due to the cholera vibrio. It is characterized by a vast watery diarrhoea leading to dehydration of the patient and for most of its victims death within a day.

Cholera is not now a menace where safe water supplies exist. It will travel like a prairie fire among primitive communities using communal water supplies contaminated by the excreta of sufferers. The social consequences in Europe are negligible. In mass pilgrimages and similar groupings under tropical and sub-tropical conditions, particularly where religious and social customs clash with western ideals of hygiene, the disease can spread rapidly. It is now possible to achieve control by immediate chlorination or boiling of drinking water followed by the permanent provision of safe water and the institution of efficient personal and food hygiene measures and by health education finally supplemented by mass immunization.

Pulmonary tuberculosis is a world-wide hazard. In western countries it is decreasing owing to better medico-social conditions.

Elsewhere overcrowding in the presence of excretors, malnutrition, poor health services and ignorance combine to maintain the mass attack on the populace.

Prevention and notification of infectious disease

Legal powers exist all over the world to a greater or lesser extent to prevent the spread of epidemic, endemic, infectious disease. Special attention is paid to the danger to public health from sea and air travel.

The purpose of notifying the occurrence of certain infectious diseases to a community health officer or adviser is to:

1. Ensure the initiation of control procedures, including the tracing of contacts.
2. Allow complete investigation and surveillance of all the circumstances.
3. Enable records to be made. The success of statutory control measures and immunization programmes can be determined only by the incidence of the specific infectious diseases.

Family doctors, heads of households and persons in charge of premises are required to send to the community health adviser a certificate notifying the occurrence of certain prescribed infectious diseases.

Some of the provisions for preventing the spread of disease can be as follows:

1. Anyone knowing that he is suffering from a notifiable disease exposes other persons to the risk of infection by his presence or conduct in any street, public place, place of entertainment or assembly, club, hotel, inn or shop, or being in charge of such an infected person allows him to conduct himself similarly, is liable to a fine.
2. The same applies to a person who gives, lends, sells, transmits or exposes without previous disinfection any clothing, bedding, or any other article, which he knows has been exposed to infectious disease.
3. Persons who suffer from infectious disease must not carry on an occupation which is a danger to others. A child may not attend school unless certain safeguards are observed.

4. It can be an offence to send or take infected linen to a laundry or public wash-house. The expense of disinfecting the articles may be paid for by the public health authority.
5. Home work may be restricted on infected premises. This is contract work by skilled individuals such as seamstresses, who undertake work in their own houses.
6. Fomites can be controlled by restrictions on persons collecting or dealing in rags, old clothes, and similar articles. The circulation of potentially infected library books is prohibited. Infectious matter may not be placed in dustbins. There are infectious disease provisions about the letting and occupation of premises.

Diseases notifiable to the Medical Officer of Health (England and Wales)
(Health Services and Public Health Act 1968).

Acute encephalitis	Ophthalmia neonatorum
Acute meningitis	Paratyphoid fever
Acute poliomyelitis	Plague
Anthrax	Relapsing fever
Cholera	Scarlet fever
Diphtheria	Smallpox
Dysentery	Tetanus
(amoebic or bacillary)	Tuberculosis
Infective jaundice	Typhoid fever
Leprosy	Typhus
Leptospirosis	Whooping-cough
Malaria	Yellow fever
Measles	

Parasites

Personal infestation by parasites may cause discomfort, disability or disease.

The mode of infestation and the site are usually specific to the parasite which may attack the skin, the intestinal tract or the tissues elsewhere. Some parasites are universal, others are limited by climatic or other physical factors. Their occurrence also depends upon the way of life of the local community.

In considering infestation tropical parasitology undoubtedly takes first place. There is a great variety of infestations. It must not be forgotten that visiting Europeans are exposed to the same hazards and may show the effects after return to their own country.

Lice, fleas and bed-bugs occur everywhere. They are associated with lack of hygiene: all can carry disease. Lice are associated with typhus, fleas with plague and bugs with rickettsial disease. The three varieties of lice are the head-louse, the body-louse and the crab-louse. They are transmitted by close contact.

The importance of the louse is the potential risk of typhus and the persistence of infestation under conditions of hygiene neglect. In this connexion it should be recalled that the elaborate coiffures of eighteenth-century women were riddled with lice and that the contemporary practice of cropping or shaving the head of men who then wore wigs was to eliminate infestation. This problem of head-lice is once more increasing in significance in Britain among the least intelligent part of the community, who demand and then neglect elaborate styles of hairdressing.

Lice go with poverty, disrupted life and war.

Control has been greatly eased by the introduction of the newer chemicals, notably DDT which can be applied successfully by dusting and spraying. Such simple action benefits the community by the abolition of the irritation which in turn leads to lack of rest and sleep and so reduces the efficiency of workman, housewife and schoolchild alike.

The same problem of inefficiency from loss of rest applies to infestation by fleas. Fleas are the vector of plague. Under suitable circumstances they are an immediate potential hazard as soon as the infection appears.

The essential action both socially and as a matter of hygiene is prevention, that is the elimination of infestation.

Bed-bugs are a social menace as they can make dwellings almost uninhabitable. They are extremely difficult to get rid of and call for the most vigorous measures. Their control is now possible with the new insecticides. Both fleas and bugs are killed by 'Gammexane'.

There are many varieties of mosquito. The most significant to man are the anophelines in which the female acts as carrier and intermediate host for the malaria parasite. The Culicine group can carry Filaria while *Aedes egypti* carries yellow fever. There are thirty-two native British varieties of mosquito, twenty-eight Anopheles and four Culicine. Though indigenous malaria 'ague' was common in former times it disappeared from the surviving pockets in the

Fens at the beginning of this century. There is no modern evidence of successful infection of indigenous British mosquitoes from the blood of travellers returning infected with malaria from abroad. *Culex molestans* which flourishes in certain parts of the South Coast of England is a vicious biter causing an irritant reaction with a liability to sepsis. In the past this mosquito has made houses uninhabitable. In some parts of the world, notably the Canadian seaboard, North Scotland and Norway, mosquitoes are a constant nuisance due to the irritation of their myriad bites. Mosquito control is effected by eliminating the breeding places and by the use of DDT.

There are mites specific to most major foods and many varieties of plant and animal. These mites contaminate food which then has to be destroyed. They also disturb the handling of food either by causing irritation in dockers who move the cargo or by attack on food-handlers. In addition to these special mites there is the *Sarcoptes scabei*, the itch-mite of scabies whose transmission is by the closest personal contacts as in overcrowded slums and camps.

Mites can carry disease, notable *Tsutsugamusi*, a virus disease transmitted by red mites found in the ears of rats who live in the top of coconut palms and feed on the nuts. The disease is found in the East. It can run a severe course with a fatal result. African tick typhus and relapsing fever are both carried by ticks.

Many other insects are involved in the social aspect of disease. Their importance is their ultimate effect on the local community. Trypanosomiasis (sleepy-sickness) was spread across Central Africa by infected carriers among the native porters who made up Stanley's relief expedition to find Livingstone. The vector, the tsetse fly, was present and was ready to be infected. As a result of the spread of Trypanosomiasis mass emigration or even compulsory evacuation of local African populations have occurred either to escape infection or to permit the disinfestation of local belts of tsetse fly.

Fungus disease can invade the skin as well as other organs. The commonest infection is epidermophytosis of the foot, hands, nails, and groin. 'Ringworm' in its various forms is a disappearing disease in Britain and school epidemics are a thing of the past. Actinomycosis, formerly a chronic and incurable infection of the intestinal tract, has fallen to antibiotic therapy.

Epidermophytosis is infectious and is spread by congregation in public baths and other places with wet floors. If fissures occur in the skin secondary infection takes place with consequent disability. The inconvenience of this chronic condition far outweighs its purely clinical significance.

Monilia or thrush attacks the intestinal tract of infants, causing local sepsis. In debilitated infants it may spread to the lungs, in which case it may be fatal.

The majority of worms settle in the bowel though many penetrate other tissues and infest other organs.

Hookworm is a gross economic and social parasite on already poor economies. It has been known since the time of the Pharaohs. A cycle of infection is kept up by faecal soiling of the ground and resultant penetration of the bare feet by emerging larvae.

The 'poor white' communities of the Tennessee Valley in the United States were rehabilitated a generation ago by mass treatment combined with improvement in the design of privies. There was an immediate reduction in anaemic debility, which permitted a better standard of work. This caused improvement in the communal economy and made it possible for the people to afford shoes which in turn gave protection against infestation by the penetration of the feet by larvae. Faecal contamination of the underground workings caused hookworm to become an occupational disease of Cornish tin miners and of those driving the early rail tunnels through the Alps. It is said that a hundred million people throughout the world suffer from hookworm debility.

Another disease which affects millions is schistosomiasis. There are three types, *S. japonicum* in the Far East, *S. mansoni* down the east side of Africa and in South America, and *S. haematobium* which occurs all over Africa and notably in Egypt where ancient papyri associate the infection with bathing. It is an ironic tragedy that the creation of giant modern irrigation works in Egypt as an economic measure have so spread the opportunities of infection that at least half the population have become infected in the present century. The Egyptian peasant 'fellahin' economy operates at a survival level and the measures designed to give an opportunity for a better life have made things worse. Continued neglect of or lack of treatment for schistosomiasis may lead to cancer of the bladder or rectum.

Helminth infestation. Helminth infestation in Britain is limited in general to the threadworm, *Oxyuris vermicularis*, infesting children and the unhygienic adults of the same household.

The standard of meat inspection throughout the country is such that *Taenia solium* in pork and *Taenia saginata* in beef are marginal hazards although in recent years a greater proportion of cattle is found to be infested with *Cystircercus bovis* on examination. Most cases of human infestation by *Cystircercus bovis* are detected when there is an onset of epilepsy in adult life after returning from the tropics. The fish tape-worm, *Dibothriocephalus latus*, is a curiosity only to be kept in mind. In the Midlands during the Hitler War an epidemic of *Trichinella spiralis* brought to light the habit of eating raw sausage meat.

Ascaris lumbricoides and, very rarely, *Fasciola hepatica* may be discovered in country people. The hookworm is a world-wide medico-social menace: *necator americanus* does not occur in Britain but at the end of the last century *Ankylostoma duodenale* was demonstrated as the cause of the occupational anaemia of the miners in the then flourishing Cornish tin mines.

Although the risks in this country are negligible compared with the almost universal infestation of tropical populations the hazard in the human relation with the alternative hosts must always be recalled as a possibility. Recent work has shown that there may be some relationship with blindness, particularly in children, by infestation with the larval form of the dog roundworm, *Toxocara canis*. Careful epidemiological studies will, no doubt, reveal other hitherto unsuspected risks.

10

Water

WATER is the prime essential for life. An adequate supply of pure water is the most elementary and important community health measure.

Water-borne infectious disease is the commonest community hazard throughout the world. Safe drinking water removes this risk. An adequate water supply permits personal cleanliness and at once helps the promotion of hygienic food handling and reduces the risk of food-poisoning. It becomes possible to launder clothing, to wash and cleanse dwellings, to operate abattoirs, dairies and adequate food premises and to promote street cleansing, water-carriage sanitation and an adequate sewerage system.

The fortunate circumstances of Britain and the more densely populated areas of Europe and North America include adequate piped supplies of pure water. Elsewhere and particularly in the less developed countries of the world water supplies may be inadequate in quantity and hazardous in safety and quality except where towns have been equipped with waterworks of European type.

Ultimately all drinking water is derived from rain. Rain is naturally distilled water vapour in the form of clouds which condense and fall to earth. If it passes through clear air and falls on a remote area the resulting accumulation can be regarded as safe. On the other hand, the rain may fall through a dusty or smoke-laden atmosphere when it will bring down with it some of this contamination. If the rain falls on ground polluted by animals or humans it is no longer safe. Rain falling on remote uplands runs downhill to form streams and rivers making their way to the sea or to a lake and liable to contamination in the process.

Various inorganic and organic salts are taken up into solution. An extreme example is the way in which water falling on a peat bog becomes acid in reaction and tinted by organic material. Water can be drawn off for use as a community supply at any point in the everlasting cycle from rain to the sea.

Rainwater can be collected from the roof for use in an individual house. The water is stored in barrels or preferably in covered

underground tanks. There must be sufficient water to provide an
adequate reserve supply. The normal practice is to provide house
tanks for one thousand gallons based on a personal consumption
of five gallons per head.

Roof collection is of use only where isolation and the absence
of better facilities make it necessary. Other methods must be
employed to provide a community supply.

Upland rain-water falling on rock can be collected either in a
lake or reservoir. If the water is to be used for human consumption measures against pollution must be taken including the control
of farms and indiscriminate access to the lake shore. In recent
years there has been a tendency to relax controls as a reasonable
degree of purity is achieved by the isolation of the site. Reservoir
water of this sort is self purifying if left for a period of a month.

Water taken from streams and rivers must always be regarded
as polluted though isolated and inaccessible rivers are self purifying
much in the same way as are the lakes.

In a few remote places in the world seawater is distilled for
drinking water. The process is quite uneconomic by ordinary
standards and the community must have some special reason for
its continued existence to justify such an arrangement.

When rain soaks into the ground it can be recovered from
shallow wells, from *deep* wells or from *Artesian* wells. It also re-
appears on the surface by the action of *springs* which may be
seasonal, intermittent or *constant*.

The subsoil is saturated by the rain which penetrates downwards
until it meets the first water-resistant stratum. It is possible to
sink shallow wells to tap the local accumulation of water. This
water has not had the benefit of any effective filtering action by the
earth. There is always a hazard from the pollution of the soil by
accumulation of filth, by manure heaps and by badly conducted
privies or cracked and leaking cesspools. There is an additional
risk from contamination by material falling or being kicked into
the well and from the traffic around the well mouth.

To cut down the risk the brick lining of the well is continued
upwards from the surface of the water to about two feet above
ground level. An impervious paving about six feet wide is laid
round the well.

A shallow well must not be within 50 feet of a dwelling house
and not within 100 feet of a privy or similar hazard.

Water is recovered from a shallow well either by the traditional

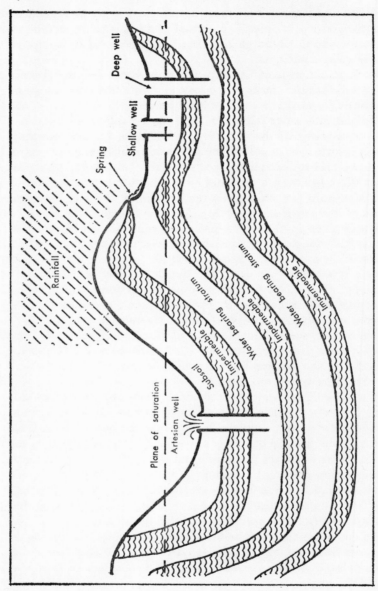

Water-supplies (wells, etc.)

bucket and windlass or by means of a pump. The bucket used must be permanently attached to the well-rope or chain and must be kept clean. The well should have a close-fitting hinged lid for cleanliness and easy access. If a pump is used it may be a hand worked suction pump, a modern semi-rotary pump or a mechanically propelled pump. The water can be delivered directly into buckets or it may be pumped into a tank for local gravity supply.

A shallow well is usually only sufficient to supply a group of buildings or a hamlet. The water is always suspect. In addition to the risk of bacteriological pollution there is always a hazard, particularly to small children, from the presence of nitrites due to pollution by organic matter. The water supply from shallow wells is directly proportionate to the local rainfall. They are seasonal, they have a limited output and in time of drought can fail completely.

Deep wells take water from underground accumulated in strata of chalk, sandstone and soft rock which acts as a huge sponge. The water can be tapped, preferably beneath an impermeable stratum, by a simple well shaft or, more efficiently, by the driving of radial horizontal tunnels called *adits* from the well shaft. These provide a greater area of exposed surface from which the water can seep into the well. As many geological strata have cracks or fissures, underground streams occur. These can be tapped and so directly increase the capacity of the deep well.

Purity is generally assured by the action of filtration through porous strata. Advantage may be taken of the flow of water through horizontal fissures but vertical fissures are a menace as they permit the direct ingress into the depths of contaminated surface water and so imperil one of the main advantages of the use of deep wells, namely freedom from pollution.

Geological strata are only theoretically horizontal. Where they *dip* or slope water will run down on top of the impervious layers just as on the surface. When the folds form a subterranean bowl, water will accumulate below ground in this depression. Sometimes the underground depression becomes overfull. The water is then under pressure. If a natural fissure or crack opens on the surface the water is forced up and escapes as a *spring*. Water restrained under pressure in these conditions can be tapped by an *Artesian well* in which the water is forced to the surface without mechanical means. It is an artificial spring. Such accumulations of water can be too *freely* tapped as in the case of the Thames Valley

in and around London to such a degree that the Artesian phenomenon is permanently diminished and the *water-table* or level
of the water below the surface falls and is only partially
restored.

The water of rivulets and streams is subject to the same pollution as that from shallow wells. River water can be freely used as
a supply provided that there is no gross chemical pollution and that
adequate filtration and purification plant is provided. The amount
of water taken from a river is limited by law. A certain amount
called 'compensation water' must be allowed to flow on for the use
of people downstream. There are stringent measures of legal control
over pollution hazards from noxious substances. Rivers, if left alone
are self purifying by a combined process of dilution, oxidation,
sedimentation, the action of water animals and plant life and sun-
light.

Distribution of water

It is rare that a source of upland water can be immediately connected to a distribution system. The water is first accumulated in
bulk in a reservoir. This may be a natural lake, a lake that has been
modified for the task, a valley blocked by a dam at its lower end or
an artificially constructed reservoir.

By the use of such *storage reservoirs* water is made available
irrespective of changing seasonal and climatic conditions. The
usual capacity provided is 100 days' water supply at normal consumption rates. Storage reservoirs are sited conveniently for the
accumulation of water and may be many miles away from the community supplied. The water is brought by one or more large pipes
or aqueducts to a purification plant where the water is treated to
make it bacteriologically pure. It is then fed into the service reservoirs and so into the distribution system for the area to be served.
This subdivides into units for convenient local connexions to
streets and individual premises. A simple system, if allowed to
expand, would branch out in the same way as a tree. Such an
arrangement leads to *stasis* which is undesirable. Wherever possible
a modern system employs a ring arrangement of main service
water pipes so that the bulk of water is kept moving and to reduce
the number of dead ends to the minimum. Stasis leads to the
accumulation of rust and occasionally of chlorine so that when the
water is allowed to flow after standing for a period there is an

unpleasant initial flow of discoloured water possibly with chlorine detectable by odour or even taste.

Local supply is by gravity from a minor service reservoir through service mains to a point nearest the premises where the *private* service pipe is connected. This is brought to a *stop-cock* which is a tap provided to control or shut off the individual supply. The supply of water from local service reservoirs is so planned that under normal conditions the pressure or *head* of water will lift it twenty feet above the roof of the premises served to facilitate fire-fighting.

Distribution of water is normally *constant*. In some areas either because of inadequacy of the equipment or of shortage of water an *intermittent* supply is provided. This is undesirable as it means that gravity storage tanks have to be provided in houses. These are always liable to be a source of pollution and plumbing trouble. The interruption of the supply causes negative pressure in the supply pipes with a potential hazard of drawing in contaminated water or other material from outside the system. An intermittent supply prevents the use of automatic sanitary flushing systems and also the washing down of premises when convenient. If a fire occurs the intermittent supply has to be re-connected forthwith.

Problems can arise in any distribution system. If iron pipes are used, the formation of rust leads to intermittent discoloration of the water, particularly when engineering work has to be done. Some waters, particularly soft waters with an acid content, are plumbo-solvent. Those who consume such water are exposed to the risk of chronic lead poisoning. Copper supply pipes may give rise to anxiety when they are new and the interior has not yet developed a surface film. Traces of the new copper are taken up by the chlorinated water and carried into kettles with subsequent formation of and discoloration from verdigris.

Domestic gravity storage tanks must be kept covered to avoid the ingress of foreign matter. They should be cleaned out at intervals. These tanks are apt to rust and so cause discoloration of the domestic hot water supply.

Chlorinated water acts as an electrolyte and under suitable conditions of metallic contrast can cause taps and metallic parts of sanitary flush tanks to become eroded and so rendered useless.

In some rural and less developed areas water is not conveyed inside the building but is brought outside either to a standpipe serving several dwellings or to an external tap outside the individual house. Water is drawn off as required and is carried indoors. The usual reason for this practice is that there is no drainage system and therefore no means of getting rid of any large bulk of water which would be introduced into the house by the installation of taps to sinks, washbasins and a bath.

When water is carried the consumption is reckoned to be five gallons per head a day. When a constant piped supply is used the consumption rises to fifty gallons per head a day. Figures vary but show a constant increase in consumption as living standards rise.

Drinking water	0.5 gallon
Cooking, personal washing... ...	5 gallons
W.C.	5 gallons
Laundry, kitchen and domestic use	10 gallons
Domestic bath	30 gallons
Horse	15 gallons
Cow	10 gallons
Hospital (per person)	50 gallons
Offices	10 gallons
Day Schools	10 gallons
Municipal Services	5 gallons

In theory it is necessary to purify only drinking water, water for washing the teeth and water for surgical procedures. Only under extreme circumstances is such a policy adopted. To have two supplies, one pure and one contaminated, is to run all the risks associated with confusion of origin by children and others not familiar with such a complex arrangement. All water supplies are fully purified whenever possible.

Boiling purifies water but this is possible only in the case of water used for personal domestic purposes or for individual household action in the face of a water-borne epidemic due to a polluted community supply.

It is more than possible that the inhabitants of rural China have survived the constant and widespread national hazard of major water-borne epidemics only by the universal habit of drinking tea. Herodotus records that in the classical pre-Christian era the Emperor of the Persians, when travelling, drank only boiled water which was carried on the journey in covered silver vessels.

Chemical treatment of water can be given by *chlorine* in the shape of bleaching powder or hypochlorite added till free chlorine exists in excess at the level of 1 part per million. After standing for half an hour sodium thiosulphate is introduced to neutralize the free chlorine. Proprietary systems employing suitable tablets are used by armies in the field and by expeditions. *Potassium permanganate* can be used: it is added in watery solution to promote mixing: to be effective the pink colour should persist for half an hour.

Precipitation and *filtration* may be used to *clarify* water but is of no value in securing a bacteriologically safe water supply unless complex and expensive apparatus is available as in modern army water purification vehicles.

Distillation of an unsafe or undrinkable water will produce a safe supply. Such a water must be aerated to make it reasonably pleasant to drink. Chemically, it is too soft and can be plumbo-solvent.

Large scale purification of water

The removal of organic pollution is achieved by storage, by filtration and by sterilization.

Storage for three or four weeks causes a marked reduction in bacteriological pollution. At the same time it permits the growth of algae which may make the water unpleasant in taste or smell. This can be prevented by the addition of copper sulphate at a rate of ten pounds per million gallons of water. The distribution in the reservoir must be carried out evenly and systematically. Objectionable taste can be got rid of by the addition of activated charcoal at the rate of ten parts per million. The charcoal is subsequently extracted at the filters.

Large scale filtration is almost universally done by the use of sand filters. These are usually slow sand filter beds with a water capacity of two gallons per square foot per hour. They can be speeded up by preliminary rapid mechanical filtration at the rate of 100 gallons per square foot per hour which is designed to remove coarser organic matter.

A slow filter depends upon the formation of an algal gel on the surface. The efficiency of the filtration is governed by the thickness of this organic pellicle. It becomes inefficient and is removed every six weeks or so and reforms after three days. In the interval the water is run through very slowly or is permitted to run to waste. For continuous working a battery of filters must operate in rotation.

Mechanical filters do not have this biological film and therefore must rely on a flocculant coagulation of aluminium sulphate to coat the filter surface. Mechanical filters can be fed by gravity or under pressure. Because of their much greater capacity for a given area mechanical filters may be used instead of slow sand filters in order to save space.

Sterilization of water in bulk is achieved by the addition of a chemical agent which destroys pathogenic bacteria. The commonest process is chlorination. Chlorine is effective in low concentration. It can be added as bleaching powder, as hypochlorite or in modern waterworks practice by using chlorine stored in liquid form in cylinders and released as gas by an automatic apparatus.

Bleaching Powder is added at the rate of 66 grains per ton of water (220 gallons) to achieve a concentration of 1 part per million. The dry powder is worked up into a paste with water and then mixed with sufficient volume of water to make it convenient to mix with the main bulk of water. Normally a concentration of 0·25 parts per million will be necessary for a filtered water. This needs about eight pounds of bleaching powder or two and a half pounds of liquid chlorine for every million gallons of water. This process is primitive but effective for small quantities of water. It is not suitable for bulk sterilization of a constant flow of water.

Various substances including vegetable matter and iron take up a great deal of chlorine by oxidation. For this reason accurate sterilization is only possible by the chlorination of water filtered to reduce oxidizable material to a minimum. The time of exposure to the chlorine is important and a period of two to four hours is not unreasonable.

When traces of phenols from road washings and other sources are present chlorination will produce an unpleasant taste. This phenomenon can be reduced by the use of chloramination which means the simultaneous addition of chlorine and ammonia. This process is less affected by organic matter than is chlorination. Exposure must be longer to achieve sterilization and much greater quantities of chemicals are used.

Breakpoint Chlorination consists of the accurate addition of a sufficient quantity of chlorine to oxidize all the ammonia present and to leave a small residuum of the chlorine.

Ozonodization is the sterilization of filtered water by exposure to *ozone*, which releases its third atom of oxygen and becomes O_2. Ozone is generated by the discharge of a high tension current across spark gaps in air. The mixture of gases is passed through water in a tower in order to achieve full mixing.

Other methods of sterilization which have not achieved great popularity are the use of excess lime, ultra violet light or the Catadyn process employing activated silver.

Hardness in water

There are two forms of hardness in water, permanent hardness due to the presence of calcium and magnesium sulphates and temporary hardness due to calcium and magnesium bicarbonates.

Hardness is a disadvantage as it causes deposits in boilers and pipes. This, in turn, can cause obstruction and local overheating with risk of explosion: it is wasteful of soap and reduces lathering: it hinders and causes curd in laundry processes: hard water is not as good as soft water for horticulture.

Temporary hardness is most evident in the 'furring' of kettles and the formation of excessive scum on the surface of used bath water. Temporary hardness can be removed by boiling or by the addition of excess of lime whereby the bicarbonates are converted into insoluble carbonates which can be filtered off.

Permanent hardness is removed by the addition of caustic soda or soda with the formation of the inert sodium sulphate.

Water softeners work on the principle of base exchange whereby the sodium in the soda/aluminium silicate complex is replaced by the magnesium and calcium drawn from the hard water: these two metals are displaced by sodium once more when the filter is regenerated by the passage of a strong solution of common salt (NaCl).

It is undesirable to use the base exchange system in the presence of lead pipes as these may become eroded. The erosion can be prevented by by-passing a certain amount of untreated hard water so that a moderate degree of hardness persists.

Water-borne disease

Water-borne disease is of special significance as it is associated with the essential need for drinking water and because consumption of affected water by the community will lead to an epidemic.

Inorganic salts can cause trouble: excessive amounts of sulphates can cause diarrhoea: the presence of lead or other metals can lead to chronic poisoning. The absence of iodine is associated with goitre: the presence of fluorine protects the teeth.

Harmful parasites can be ingested such as bilharzia, filaria, hookworm, guinea worm, flukes, oxyuris and ascaris.

Pathogenic bacteria are the most significant risk. These include typhoid, paratyphoid, cholera and the dysenteries. In the quarter of a century which ended in 1937 over twenty major outbreaks of typhoid occurred in Britain due to the contamination of a public water supply. There are rules of conduct for water undertakings and it is only when these are ignored or broken that trouble starts.

It is appropriate to mention that the water supply of merchant ships normally depends upon tanks replenished from the public supply at ports of call. Water-borne disease in these circumstances is exceedingly rare and yet it is commonplace to blame the ship's water supply for the outbreaks of gastro-enteritis which frequently occur in passenger ships. These are really food poisoning episodes due to the lack of cleanliness and hand hygiene among the ship's catering staff. A moment of reflection would allay much anxiety when it is realized that the patients are associated only with certain localized feeding arrangements in the ship. Other groups fed from other sources are not affected. If the water-supply of the vessel were the cause then all on board would be equally affected.

Ice is water in another physical state. If the original water had been bacteriologically polluted then this pollution remains, controlled only by the process of freezing. If ingested with or reconstituted as water and consumed the appropriate pathological manifestation will occur.

Analysis of water

The chemical analysis of water is confined to the details of hardness, of trace elements such as fluorine, the presence of special inorganic constituents of which the salt of seawater are an example and the chemical evidence of organic pollution as demonstrated by the presence of nitrates and nitrites.

The more significant analysis is bacteriological and for all practical purposes is related to the hazard of pathogenic bowel-borne bacteria present either by direct contamination or by the entry of sewer contents into the water supply. The direct identification of pathogenic bacteria in a large number of routine samples would be an uneconomic and impracticable operation in terms of skilled time expended and the apparatus and materials involved.

The universal bacterium in the human bowel is *E. coli faecalis*. It is sufficient to demonstrate its presence to infer that there is a hazard from faecal contamination and therefore a potential health hazard which becomes real if the faecal contamination involves a carrier of bowel-borne disease in general and typhoid in particular.

E. coli faecalis in raw water must be eliminated by chlorination or comparable treatment. If *E. coli* is recovered from a treated water then the treatment is ineffective and must be given attention forthwith.

The present-day supply of water by large-scale water undertakings is a civil engineering project carried out by skilled specialist staff. While there must always be a final medical responsibility for the safety of the water supply this is normally exercised indirectly. Standards are set out which correspond to normal good water practice: there is then only the necessity to keep the medical officer informed of anything that appears to be amiss, of any new project or of any major alterations or repairs to the system.

In this connexion it is necessary to mention that workpeople who are in a position accidentally to contaminate the supply should all be medically examined for freedom from being carriers of bowel borne disease. It was this failure together with the fouling of one of the deep wells which led to the great typhoid epidemic at Croydon in 1937.

The purity and adequacy of a water supply must be checked from time to time. Since the water is supplied to every area in a community, a danger to health arises from any inadequacy or impurity of the supply. A community may supply water to premises outside their own area or supply an adjoining district in bulk.

Communities have to provide waterworks. Before a major reservoir is contructed, notice has to be given so that local objectors may have their complaints examined. The community must have powers to lay and maintain water mains. Public wells, pumps and other apparatus for the provision of an adequate supply of water to the inhabitants have to be tested and kept under the control of the community. A charge or rate may be levied for the provision of water.

The community should see that both new dwellings and houses already occupied are provided with a sufficient water supply. The community must have powers to prohibit or restrict the use of water from a polluted supply. In this connexion a well, tank, cistern or water-butt used for the supply of water for domestic purposes which is so placed, constructed or kept as to render the water liable to contamination prejudicial to health is held to be a nuisance.

I I

Sewage Disposal

KNOWLEDGE that human excreta can be a vehicle for the transmission of disease is traditional in many racial and religious cultures. Often cultural customs aid public health by postulating some standard method of disposal. Scientific knowledge of the hazards make it even more compelling that the community should not be put to unnecessary risk. The method of disposal adopted must be efficient and reliable or the end result will be worse than the beginning.

Sewage consists of solid and liquid human excreta and, in addition, waste water from dwelling houses, trade wastes and rainwater, surface water and road-washings.

The consistency of sewage varies with its water content. When water is taken into a house it has to be got out again. The personal carriage of water from a well or standpipe restricts the use of water to small quantities which set no problem in disposal. Piped water lends to liberal use in sinks, washbasins and baths, thus making it imperative to have some drainage system for eventual removal. This makes it possible to have a water-carriage system of sewage disposal. The waste water acts as a vehicle for the carriage of solid excreta. The provision of water closets requires a further supply of water for their operation. In general it is the quantity of sewage which determines the method of disposal and this is linked with the average water consumption per head of the local population. Where there is no piped water supply to houses then dry or *conservancy* methods of disposal of excreta are used: where there is a liberal water supply a *drainage* system must be provided. The contrast is evident when it is realized that without a piped water supply the average daily consumption of water is about five gallons per head: with a piped water supply the figure is around fifty gallons per head. A convenient calculation of the excreta involved is made at the rate of 4 oz. of faeces and 40 oz. of urine per person per day.

If it is not possible to provide a proper sewage scheme then human excreta must be kept and then removed in bulk at frequent

95

intervals. In addition, some method of dealing with waste water must be arranged.

In conservancy disposal *pail closets* and *earth closets* are the most suitable appliance for use when the contents are to be disposed of on dry land. In all cases the pail or container used must be watertight and impervious. If the closet is to be used merely as a receptacle then it is known as a *pail closet*. It has to be kept covered and flyproof and emptied frequently to prevent nuisance. As a refinement dry earth or ash can be used as a deodorizer and will aid the disintegration of the faeces. By its use a less distasteful method of disposal can be achieved. A stock of dried earth is provided for the user to scatter over and cover the excrement on leaving. The container stands in a box with the top formed into a seat and covered by a close-fitting lid. This *earth closet* should be fly-proofed in the same way as the pail closet and both must be emptied with the most careful attention to cleanliness. The drier the process the less is the offence and the easier the disposal. Waste water must be excluded. The pail contents can be disposed of by trenching in land, by incineration or by composting with dry refuse. The risk of conserving treatment is associated with the disposal of excreta from patients and carriers of typhoid and other bowel complaints. The threat to shallow wells should not be ignored. Though the process appears so simple as to be of little cost a further examination of the expense of cart collection will show that in a bigger area there is very little difference between conservancy and water-carriage systems over a long period. With a conservancy system there must be a separate arrangement for removing waste either into a soakaway, on to a garden or in a more organized way by running a series of agricultural drains at a suitable depth under a plot of land or a tilled part of the garden.

A *chemical closet* is a container appliance fitted with a seat and lid and in which the excreta is received into a disinfectant and deodorant solution. The liquid is either an alkaline emulsion of coal tar or a strong solution of caustic soda. Disinfection of the solids is not always complete. Disposal is usually by burial. The method is suitable for isolated dwellings or for temporary use where portability is especially desirable.

The *bore-hole latrine* is a simple device common in the tropics and often used for temporary installations in Europe. It has the advantage that there is no fly problem. It consists of a round hole of varying size from nine inches to sixteen inches in diameter

bored out with a special auger to a depth of twelve to twenty feet.
The top is fitted either with a pair of concrete slabs as footrests on
which the user can squat or for European use with a conventional
seat. The latrine can be used for long periods without attention and
there appears to be relatively little risk to water supplies.

A *cesspool* is essentially an underground watertight tank for the
reception of sewage. Cesspools are constructed of rendered brick.
They are covered and are provided with a means of access and an
effective method of ventilation. The drain from the house is led to
the cesspool. Rainwater is deflected into soakaways in order to
reduce the bulk of sewage.

There is no special process associated with a cesspool. It is
simply a bulk storage for sewage which has to be emptied at
frequent intervals. A cesspool rarely remains sound. A leaking
cesspool can contaminate a drinking-water supply. The cesspool
should never be sited less than a hundred feet from a well or fifty
feet from a house.

A *water-carriage* system of sewage disposal depends upon a
liberal water supply with appropriate arrangements for the removal
of waste water through drains and sewers. A *drain* is used for the
drainage of one set of premises: a *sewer* is part of the general
system of removal from a number of premises and is the channel to
which the individual drains are connected as tributaries.

To retain their contents drainpipes must be impervious and so
are usually made of cast-iron or of glazed-clay. Unglazed clay-pipes
and earthenware are unsuitable for use in sanitary work. They are
used only for agricultural drainage where their texture allows
gradual percolation of the contents into the soil.

A drain has to work automatically without becoming blocked or
otherwise causing inconvenience or nuisance. The drain must be
self-cleansing by the scouring action of its contents. This is
effected by the careful laying of the drain in straight lines or easy
bends, by the smoothness of the interior lining and by the use of a
suitable gradient, or *fall*, to ensure a proper velocity and depth of
flow to make the contents truly waterborne. The junctions and
other places where drain stoppage may occur must be accessible for
attention. The whole system must be ventilated to prevent the
accumulation of foul air. All drain outlets are sealed by a simple
contrivance called a trap working on the same principle as the
familiar S-shaped device under the outlet of a washbasin. The
working of the seals of the traps relies on the maintenance of a

H

pocket of water in the base of the trap to submerge the communicating openings and so prevent the passage of foul gas.

A sewerage system must be laid in a similar way so that it will not become blocked. As petrol and oil are nowadays in such common use the risk of their accidental admission to a sewer is not inconsiderable with the consequent hazard of explosion or of spreading fire menacing the workmen. For this reason the sewers must be well ventilated. In times of storm and excessive rainfall the ventilation system prevents air compression in the sewer due to sudden increase in the bulk of its contents.

Sewers must be soundly constructed to prevent leakage. According to size they may be of glazed clay, concrete or built of brick. Cast iron is used only where special strength is needed. Leakage is important from the point of view of the pollution of water. Sewers are often laid in close proximity to waterpipes. If the phenomenon of *negative pressure* or suction occurs in the water mains, subsoil water is drawn in from the surrounding earth. If a nearby sewer is leaking the subsoil water will be polluted and the final result is sewage pollution of the water supply.

Water-borne sewage must be disposed of so that it does not become a menace to health. In coastal areas it can conveniently be discharged into the sea. This simple method of disposal cannot be applied to rivers, lakes and other potential sources of fresh water for drinking. Arrangements have to be made for processing the sewage. The method depends upon a final separation of the solids from the water element; the latter being eventually purified to a sufficient degree to be safely passed into a river or stream.

The first process is to have a means of coping with the sudden overloading of the system by sudden and heavy rainfall. This is done by a system of weirs which permit the excess to pass to storage or to escape directly by means of a storm overflow.

Sewage contains a variety of solid matter. This is filtered off or screened and then disposed of by burial, incineration, composting or in some instances by fermentation in closed tanks from which the resultant methane is drawn off and burnt as a source of heat or power. On its way along the sewer the sewage accumulates grit and other solid material which has to be removed at the sewage works by passage through detritus tanks or grit chambers at slow speed to permit as much detritus as possible to fall out. The major solids are removed in this way but further precipitation is effected by tank treatment. This is done by passing the sewage through long deep tanks arranged in pairs or groups for alternate use in order to permit removal of the resultant sludge.

By now the remains of the sewage is in liquid form called *tank liquor*. Tank liquor can be given *sewage farm* or *land treatment*. The liquor is run over specially reserved land into which it soaks but is not permitted to destroy the plant life. The ground thus acts as a filter. In spite of the reduction in the number of bacteria pathogenic organisms may survive. An alternative is the *biological method of treatment*. *Biological filters* are large circular filter beds of clinker or stone. The liquor is fed to the upper surface of the bed by rotating sprinkler arms. The action is a nitrifying one aided by the free access of oxygen from the air, the humidity and the warmth of fermentation. *Contact beds* work on the same principle but are less efficient.

In the *activated sludge process* the screened sewage is mixed with ripened or mature sludge and aerated so that a constant process of fermentation goes on. It works on the principle of enrichment of the fermentation process by the enhanced bacterial content of the more mature additive. The disposal of resultant sludge is a major problem as agriculturists do not always favour its use on the land.

The purification of sewage is little done in Britain. It consists of dosing the tank liquor with necessarily big doses of chlorine or its sources. A long period of contact is required. The resultant effluent is lethal to fish.

The *discharge of trade wastes into sewers* is permitted under certain controlled conditions. Irrespective of their content it is desirable for the amount admitted at any given time to be proportionate to the flow of normal sewage.

Trade wastes fall into three main groups. The first consists of those inert substances which can be removed by simple sedimentation and filtration. These include the waste from china-clay works, stone quarries, coal washing installations and the like. The second group contains polluting substances in solution and solids in suspension. These require treatment by sedimentation and chemical processes. The third group consists of polluting substances in solution or colloidal suspension as occurs when a bulk of milk is mixed with sewage. This group required chemical or biological treatment.

For small camps or isolated buildings it is the practice to install a *septic tank* designed to retain the sewage for a sufficient time to cause break-up of the solid material and to allow the insoluble matter to precipitate as sludge. The effluent is purified aerologically by means of a percolating filter or aeration bed. The resulting effluent should be fit for discharge into a stream or by irrigation. To be effective the tank must not be too big as the resulting effluent must be relatively fresh and not be decomposed. An effective capacity is rather less than one day's sewage. The effluent must pass through a humus tank for final settling immediately before it is passed into any slow-running stream to avoid local fouling.

An embarrassing complication of sewage treatment practice has been introduced by the common household use of detergents whereby excessive foam is generated at the sewage works. Quite apart from its nuisance value the foam can coat filters and so seal them off from adequate air contact. In consequence the biological action of the sewage treatment system can be hindered. The final effluent entering a stream can carry sufficient detergent to cause the unsightly appearance of foam which may be carried downstream for miles.

Sewer systems are always liable to have to cope with the spread and increase in the number of buildings they are required to serve. As a result sewers become obsolete either in capacity or in design. This may first become obvious to the casual observer when the already overtaxed sewers are exposed to the impact of heavy rainfall with consequent overloading of their carrying capacity.

Water falling on roofs and roads must be drained away. In an area with underground water supplies in chalk it is desirable to conserve every drop of rain which if it had not fallen on a roof would have fallen on the ground, soaked in and passed to the supply. This is done by arranging that all possible rainwater is diverted into soakaways and not into the drains and sewers. Road surface water is likely to be contaminated both by the content of the dust with which it is in contact and also by the traces of phenols from tar and other chemicals which it washes out from the road-making materials. Even these traces can cause unpleasant taste in drinking water after chlorination and the consequent oxidizing reaction.

If a separate system of sewers has been provided for the purpose then the admission of storm water is at once under control Such an installation is much less common than the combined system whereby one sewer takes both sewage and rain and storm water. The usual calculation is for the sewer to be big enough to take three times the normal flow. Some form of by-pass system is necessary to cope with a greater volume. The sewer may at some stage be formed as an open channel. When the level of the contents rises too high overflow occurs. This overflow is diverted into storm water tanks for disposal after the immediate emergency.

Sudden heavy rain pouring into a combined sewer system can produce such rapid increase in the bulk of sewage that the equivalent of a river 'bore' or tidal wave can be caused. In big sewers this is a recognized hazard and on occasion workmen have been engulfed.

If the whole cross-section of the sewer is filled by its contents it is said to be *supercharged*. The only relief to the pressure is for the sewer contents to rise in the manholes and to force up the lids and escape into the streets. Those drain connections where backflow constitutes a special risk as in the case of food premises can be protected from the effects of back pressure by the fitting of non-return valves. These close automatically when the flow is reversed and so prevent a disastrous backflow of sewage.

The discharge of sewage into the sea

The practice of discharging sewage into the sea is almost universal in coastal areas where it is also the most economical method of disposal.

Seaside towns and villages usually grow up at some point on the coast where a stream in a valley runs into the sea. Building follows the natural contours. The first sewers were laid in the last century before the notable expansion of resorts which occurred in the motor car age. In consequence the sewer system has of necessity to be expanded to match and has usually done so by additions to the original layout. Just as water flows to the sea the same gradients provide a natural feature aiding the sewerage system to follow a similar route.

The sewage is passed into the sea through a long pipe called an outfall, the siting and construction of which requires the careful application of civil engineering practice to local conditions. The end of the outfall must be sufficiently far out to sea and in such a position that the sewer contents will not come ashore due to the effect of wind and current.

From time to time it is suggested that the method of disposal is injurious to health from the risk due to bowel-borne infectious disease. If this argument is valid it must stand up to careful epidemiological study in relation to the whole area. Consideration has to be given to the possibility of infecting shellfish and the need to ban their collection from the foreshore. This problem must be considered in relation to its size and significance when contrasted with the need for providing convenient and economical sewage disposal for a large community.

It is not necessary to treat sewage passed into the sea except for aesthetic reasons. The main effort should be directed to removing or breaking up visible and obnoxious solid matter so that distasteful consequences are avoided.

12

Housing

DWELLINGS differ in construction according to climate and culture. They provide protection and shelter against extremes of weather, as well as privacy and facilities for a healthy and hygienic way of life.

The house must be adequate in size and accommodation and economic to run, and to rent or buy. It should be conveniently sited for community activities, for work, for schools, for shopping and for travel. Housing is a matter of compromise in siting between town and country, in the availability of sites, in the economics of size and amenity, in fitness for a modern way of life, in relation to the design, construction, age and condition of the house and the amount the occupant is willing to spend on satisfying his housing needs either by rent or by purchase, and on repair and alteration.

Today in advanced communities the housewife in all ranks of society has personal commitments about the house; there is the strongest possible case for making that part of the house worked in by the housewife and used for ordinary daytime life the sunniest and most interesting. The former idea of preserving the best rooms of the house for formal occasions is fading away under the pressure of changed social usage and the need to use all available space to the full. The objective today can be summarized by saying the house should have a kitchen with a view.

The following criteria have been laid down for a modern dwelling. It should:

1. Be in all respects dry.
2. Be in a good state of repair.
3. Have each room properly lighted and ventilated.
4. Have an adequate supply of wholesome water laid on for all purposes inside the dwelling.
5. Have an efficient and adequate hot water supply for domestic purposes.
6. Have an internal readily accessible water-closet.
7. Have a fixed bath, preferably in a separate room.

103

8. Be provided with one or more sinks and with suitable arrangements for the disposal of waste water.
9. Have facilities for domestic washing.
10. Have a proper drainage system.
11. Have adequate artificial lighting in each room.
12. Have adequate facilities for heating each habitable room.
13. Have satisfactory facilities for preparing and cooking food.
14. Have a well ventilated larder, food storage or refrigerator.
15. Have proper facilities for storage of fuel.
16. Have a satisfactory surfaced path to out-buildings, and convenient access from a street to the back door.

The house must be weatherproof. It should be impervious to damp weather through the roof, the walls, the floors and through door and window openings. The design, ventilation and construction should be such that dampness by condensation is avoided.

Houses are usually built of brick or stone but concrete and other non-traditional materials are now quite common and timber houses are coming more into use. Prefabrication in the factory of sections of a building has been introduced to speed up estate building: the practice is only really suitable for multiples of the same design of dwelling. The one advantage of brickwork is that it is the supreme flexible material: it can be laid and adjusted to any design and the result is infinitely variable. Prefabricated buildings are restricted to a small number of designs, very much like a child's toy building in which only the simplest variation of component layout is possible.

A house depends for its stability on the design, construction and siting of the foundations. Where building on rock or chalk is possible the foundations are minimal. On soft soil massive foundations on a wide base must be provided to counter any tendency to movement. Land may be reclaimed by tipping to create building sites. While it is possible to build on made-up flat sites above former rubbish tips these are always liable to be soft: they are better used for such purposes as playing fields for schools.

The foot of the outside walls of a house and those inside walls which will carry the weight of the house are expanded to double width to take the pressure from above. In some cases the house is built on an actual raft of concrete to provide support and to prevent the upward penetration of damp. Under normal circumstances the rising penetration of damp from below through the walls can be checked: to do this a damp-proof course is incorporated into the wall above the soil level but below the level of the ground floor and its supporting timbers or joists. This damp-proof course consists of a continuous strip of copper, lead sheet, asphalt or slate all round the house covering the full width or thickness of the brickwork slightly above ground level. This seals off all the structure above from the possibility of rising damp penetration by capillary action through the bricks.

Rising damp is a common feature of older houses. In some instances it can be remedied using an iso-osmotic technique. In other instances it cannot be remedied as the construction of the house does not permit of the insertion of a damp-proof course.

Floors are usually made of tongued-and-grooved planks supported on joists which rest either in niches in the walls or on a ledge contrived by the bricklayer at an appropriate height.

The space under the ground floor boards must be ventilated to prevent the growth of dry-rot (*Merulius lacrymans*) a fungus which flourishes in a still, dark, damp atmosphere.

Due to timber shortages, many modern ground floors have been made of solid concrete covered with synthetic tiles or wooden blocks often over insulating material. Solid floors are a disadvantage when underfloor plumbing and similar alterations are necessary. Unlike floor boards, solid floors are inelastic and are trying to the feet. They have the advantage that they are clean. They avoid the risk of damp and consequent dry-rot which occurs under wood floors where the space beneath is not ventilated. Solid floors are also vermin-proof.

A damp house is traditionally associated with ill health. While there is little evidence that the healthy are affected, there may be a worsening of the condition of chronic chest cases and those with a tendency to arthritis. It is probable that the indirect effect of damp is a more important threat to health. Moulds form: clothes and bedding become damp; the general conditions become uncomfortable. The main evidence of the undesirability of damp is the converse effect of its abolition and the general results of being able to live in dry conditions.

Penetrating damp makes its way in from the outside by capillary attraction and soaking. It originates either from exposure of the outside of the building to rain or a constant leak or from the moisture held in earth which is in direct contact with the affected wall. It can be stopped by making the outside of the wall waterproof. This is done by providing an external impervious protective layer or rendering, normally of cement, and by removing the offending earth.

The external walls of houses are built as cavity walls. In reality these are two thin parallel detached walls linked only at the major openings and by strengthening irons to aid stability. They have an air-space or cavity between them. This space provides a barrier to the penetration of damp and also insulation which prevents heat transfer in either direction. The insulating effect keeps the house at a more equable temperature throughout the year.

Damp may enter a house by the openings. Windows and doors wear and warp with the passage of years and so cease to be weather-proof. The design may be satisfactory under ordinary conditions and the condition of the fittings may he good but in exposed sites on hills and coasts these may fail to stand up to the extra stress either by direct failure of function or by inadequate protection being worked into the design. A visit to a place with extremes of weather will at once indicate the direction and strength of the prevailing wind not only by its bending effect on bushes and shrubs but also by the appearance of a variety of makeshift porches and similar forms of protection obviously added to houses as an after-thought to cope with inclement weather conditions.

The greatest confusion with regard to damp in houses is the occurrence of condensation. This phenomenon means that certain parts of the house are subject to the effect of the cooling of a warmer internal moisture-laden atmosphere where proper ventilation conditions do not exist, in the same way that the outside of a glass of cold water in a warm room shows condensation.

The commonest example of condensation occurs in unheated bathrooms, particularly in winter. Steam from the hot water saturates the air with water vapour which condenses to beads and then to rivulets of moisture on the windows, tiles, cold water pipes and other cool surfaces. Condensation occurs on the walls; if they are papered the moisture penetrates and soon stains and loosens the wall paper. If the walls are distempered or painted with a matt or microscopically rough surface condensation still occurs but is not immediately visible to the naked eye; it appears when the surface is touched and the droplets coalesce. If the walls are left rough plastered condensation will continue to occur in microscopic form and the droplets of moisture will soak into the plaster. If this is not soon dried out fungus spores settle and grow in the pores of the plaster, causing discoloration.

Exactly the same sort of condensation occurs in a working kitchen. It will also occur in other rooms in the house which are cold and unventilated, especially when they are used as bedrooms where the doors are closed and where sleepers introduce moisture into the atmosphere by their respiration. This situation can be much aggravated by poor design in which air circulation has been neglected, where there is an excessive proportion of outer wall in relation to the number of rooms and where there is either no open fire or central heating or these provisions are inadequate.

The situation is made worse when the exterior of the building is excessively exposed to the chilling effect of the prevailing winds, when double glazing of exposed windows has been omitted and when some novel design or construction of the building has been introduced without forethought. Under these circumstances the natural reaction of the inhabitants to condensation is to provide portable or temporary heating to combat the situation. All such heating is expensive and unfortunately the cheapest is oil heating. The burning oil at once aggravates the problem by producing water vapour as a major product of combustion. As may be expected this only contributes further to the condensation.

Roof leaks are of three types. The first is due to holes or cracks in the roof covering and can be easily traced if the roof has no lining. If there is a roof lining the penetrating rain may run down on top of the lining but below the tiles or slates. It will first show itself as a damp patch on a wall at the junction with the roof with an obvious source from above. Great patience is often needed to trace the course of the water back to its origin which may not be easily visible.

Roofs and other exposed upper surfaces have their convex angles protected by ridge tiles. Junctions of roof, chimney and walls are sealed by strips of sheet lead, zinc or copper, called flashings. These flashings are inserted under the tiles or slate and into brickwork. There is little limit to the ingenuity with which flashings can provide a watertight junction at an angle. Deterioration of the metal leads to leakage.

The third form of roof leak occurs when rain or snow is driven upwards under the tiles or slates by the wind. Moisture gains access if the angle or pitch of the slates is not steep enough to act as a barrier.

Roofs are angled or pitched except where there is a special demand for a flat roof. In contrast to slates, tiles are not completely watertight unless they are glazed on the outer surface. If fixed at a suitable angle rainwater will not penetrate completely through tiles but will tend to run downwards over the surface or within the tile itself.

A dry roof is achieved by laying tiles so that three overlap. Nothing penetrates to the third layer. As slates are inherently waterproof they only need an overlap of two.

The normal pitch of the roofs of modern British houses is 45° although variations may be seen. A number of Georgian and early Victorian houses with very flat-pitched slate roofs still exist in some localities. They appear to have been entirely successful in resisting the penetration of weathers.

Although the basic structure of a house consists of roof, walls and floors, the effective use of the house depends upon the interior details.

Houses are now usually built with two storeys of which the ground floor is used in the day and the upper floor at night. Alternatives are single floor bungalow designs and houses with three or more floors. These latter are rarely built though many thousands contructed in the last century are still put to excellent use as single dwellings or subdivided to make flats. A former practice which has almost disappeared is the provision of cellars. These make excellent storage space, boiler-rooms and coal-cellars and also create air insulation below the ground floor level.

The modern roof is lined with impervious roofing felt which is windproof as well as waterproof. When timber was cheaper it was the custom to build a complete roof lining of wood and then to secure the tiles or slates to this. By this means the roof was strengthened, made completely weathertight and considerably insulated against the loss of heat.

Heat is lost from a house through the roof by convection. It is also lost by radiation from roof, walls and windows. In addition, there is a cooling effect in the interior of the house from the cold inner surfaces of windows and walls. Cold air gains access to the house as it is drawn in both by the general convection effect and to replace air escaping from the house by reason of underdraughts in chimney flues, particularly when fires are lit. Heat loss is both undesirable and uneconomic. Any cooling effect means either that the house is more uncomfortable than it need be or that more fuel has to be burnt than is really necessary for the desired standard of warmth. The effect is of even more significance if fuel is scarce.

Heat loss can be reduced in a variety of ways. The roof itself can be insulated by the use of glass wool, aluminium foil, fibre matting, synthetic plastic or polythene foam sheets. These can be attached to the roof timbers or alternatively can be laid in the roof space to cover the ceilings of the living-rooms beneath. It must not be forgotten that if heat can no longer penetrate into the roof space the attic water tanks will need special attention and insulation to prevent them from freezing.

The spaces between ceilings and the floors above can be similarly insulated either by incorporating aluminium foil or glass matting at the time of building or by introducing some portable form of insulation into the space at a later date. Double glazing of windows is common in continental Europe where winters are harder than our own. As yet there is little provision in Britain but the practice is increasing. Cavity walls are universal; their insulating properties can be increased by using special insulating bricks for the inner brick skin or by the use of an interior insulating layer incorporated in the plaster of the room. Floors are insulated by the laying of blocks or sheets of specially designed materials. By these measures the heat loss from the house can be halved and the fullest and most economical use made of the means of heating.

Much attention is now being paid to preventing heat loss by means of insulation of lofts by fibreglass and by the double glazing of windows.

Traditionally, the English house is heated by a coal fire. This has been rightly accused of waste of heat, unneccesary smoke production and inefficiency. Inevitably, the updraught in the chimney carries off heated air as well as unconsumed fuel in powder or dust form. There is also heat loss by conduction through the actual materials of the fireplace. The open grate has been greatly improved in recent years. By attention to design a series of radiating surfaces have been contrived in the modern fireplace which direct as much heat as possible into the room. Various ingenious slow burning and other forms of grate permit the use of a greater variety of fuels with better combustion and less waste. Better chimney design aids combustion. It is possible to reduce draughts to a minimum by arranging for the essential air for combustion in the grate not to be drawn from the heated living-space but to be brought from the exterior to the fireplace through special ducts.

Fires need chimneys. According to the position of the fireplaces chimneys can be built on the outside wall of the house or rise in the interior and penetrate the roof. As the chimney itself becomes warm when fires are in use it is more economical and more comfortable when the whole of this heating effect can be used by bringing the chimneys up through the interior of the house. This is of particular benefit to the storage tanks in the roof as they can be sited near the warm brickwork of the chimney and so do not suffer the effects of frost.

Like coal fires, gas fires need a chimney or vent to remove fumes arising from combustion. From time to time attempts are made to introduce freestanding unvented gas radiators. These produce great quantities of water vapour and start or aggravate condensation problems.

Electricity is used in both fixed and portable heaters. Electric heaters are convenient and clean but relatively expensive to run. They produce a dry warmth with consequent reduction of humidity sometimes below the level of comfort. The versatility of electricity permits the incorporation of thermostatic devices and time switches so that personal needs can be met almost automatically. In addition to more conventional designs electricity can be used for overhead radiators or for under-floor heating.

The defects of any sort of individual heating unit is that it can only provide local warmth, leaving other parts of the room or house relatively cold. This deficiency may be met by space heating supplied by electric, water or steam radiators, though the latter are now obsolete. Electric radiators are expensive. Hot water radiators are the cheapest form of space heater, the operating cost depending upon the type of boiler fuel. This can be anthracite, oil, gas or, rarely, electricity. Of these, solid fuel is the cheapest, but is dusty and calls for daily stoking and frequent ash removal. Oil and gas installations are automatic and need practically no attention. They are clean and there is no dust or ash problem, but they are relatively expensive to run. Space heating is usually by a low-pressure hot water system in which heat from the boiler is exchanged into a closed hot water pipe circuit planned so that by convection it feeds radiators throughout the house and receives from them in return the cooled water which has dispersed its heat. In a home this form of heating can operate from a boiler serving the domestic hot water system.

Whenever possible radiators are placed immediately below a window to heat by convection the cold air falling from the surface of the glass.

Hot water can also be used for under-floor heating. Small-bore copper pipes are laid below the floor and hot water is forced through them by an electric pump. While the method has much to commend it, it loses the effect of simple convection and has to rely on electric power for effective circulation. Under-floor heating is for 'background' effect and must be supplemented by local heaters or fires.

To be adequate the windows of a house must be of at least one-tenth of the floor space in area. They must be so placed that they are not unduly overshadowed by adjoining structures. Some part of the window should be capable of being opened for ventilation.

Windows are of varying design. The traditional casement window which opens on hinges like a door has returned to popularity after being eclipsed for a century and a half by the sash window. The sash window, divided into upper and lower halves running in vertical grooves, is easily opened or closed as it is balanced by counterweights. Sash windows are expensive to make. Maintenance is complicated by awkward mishaps such as jamming or the breaking of the sashcords supporting the counterpoise weights. The modern casement window is made of alloy or rust-proofed steel. If it is finished accurately to engineering standards it will accept a considerable amount of misuse before it wears or distorts.

On occasion windows are made to swing on a horizontal or vertical central pivot so that the whole window area can be opened. These windows are not entirely practical and in many ways interfere with traditional furnishing and the provision of curtains. Some casement and pivot windows can be supplied with the desirable addition of double glazing as an effective measure against heat loss.

Deterioration in houses

Houses deteriorate due to neglect, age or the conduct of the residents. It must be recognized that with the growth of towns there is a tendency for those who are in a position of choice to move further away from the older obsolete centre to newer houses built to suit their needs.

The older houses are then left to be occupied by those in a lower social group. There is less spent on maintenance and less responsible behaviour. Any house if carefully maintained and left undamaged will withstand the onslaughts of extremes of weather. External woodwork should be protected by paint; doors should be rehung at the earliest signs of defect; flashings and slates should be attended to if there is any sign of leakage; gutters and down pipes need maintenance.

In the same way the interior should be kept up. Floors, staircases, walls, sanitary fittings and wiring all need periodical repair or renewal.

If maintenance is not undertaken then deterioration sets in. Windows and doors split, warp and part company at the joints. Glass becomes loose. Rain drives in and causes damp within thus making conditions worse. Window fittings rapidly deteriorate if not promptly attended to. If rainwater is allowed to pour in through an unattended roof leak ceilings begin to break up, rooms become damp and moulds and mildew flourish. When cracked or defective washbasins, water closets and sinks are left unrepaired, the people in the house change their habits of hygiene to meet the worsening conditions with an inevitable lowering of standards.

The conduct of the residents affects the situation. If they are responsible they attend to defects as they occur and so delay the effects on the fabric of the building. The feckless do nothing or even cause irresponsible damage and in consequence things get worse than they might.

The whole situation is overhung by the passage of time which brings changing social habit, changing standards and legislation, and an ageing and weakening of the building so that it becomes both obsolete and worn-out. The roof deteriorates till complete re-roofing is necessary, the walls let in damp, windows and doors need replacement: when all this and much more is remedied the house is only restored to an inferior image of what it was when new, possibly as long as a hundred years ago.

Attempts at modernization take up space not provided for when the house was designed. The end product is not unlike the amateur results of those who try to bring out-of-date motor cars to modern standards of amenity and performance.

Imperfect house maintenance proceeds under ever-worsening conditions until it appears to reach a 'point of no return' after which the property rapidly goes downhill to become a slum. This process can be prevented for many years by prudent interventive rehabilitation of houses of middle age. There are many thousands of houses about sixty years old which can be given a new and long lease of life by attention to the roof and chimneys and by bringing the interior amenities up to modern standards. The sacrifice of a bedroom converted into a bathroom and lavatory, the provision of modern grates and a hot water system, a ventilated food store and other similar items permit a higher standard of living and a reassurance that the house will not be prematurely closed or condemned as inadequate. To aid this process the community makes improvement grants based on an approved schedule of essential works.

Public health and housing laws are quite rightly designed to protect tenants from the physical consequences of the deterioration of their homes.

Dealing with defective property is a permanent and continuing responsibility of the community health adviser, whose duty it is to inspect premises and to single out those which are unfit. Thus there is progress in either remedying defects or slum clearance. The inspections are in fact carried out by community health officers, sometimes known as public health or sanitary inspectors. When defects are discovered the owner is informed. If the owner is not prepared to put things right after an informal approach then he is served with a statutory notice, which sets out a schedule of works and requires attention to them. It is the common-sense practice of certain legal systems to give anyone at fault a reasonable time to comply with requirements before penalizing him. This interim period frequently gives rise to misunderstanding as there is normally a time-lag of several weeks before enforcement is possible. Unless the reason for the delay is understood, it could be thought that the community health service was being dilatory in its duty. Action by this service is designed to remedy matters which could be a hazard to health. These consist of defects or inadequacy of the building itself, the narrowness of streets or the bad arrangements of buildings, the conduct of the residents in causing nuisance, as well as the overcrowding of rooms.

Repair of the property will not cure inherent defects such as insufficient height of rooms, the absence of, and inability to provide, a damp-proof course to check rising damp, or the absence of adequate air or light due to high adjacent buildings and other structures. When no remedy is possible at reasonable cost then the house affected should be closed as a legal requirement.

When two or more adjacent houses are affected and their defects cannot be remedied at reasonable cost, a clearance area is

I

defined. A public inquiry must be conducted if there are objectors to the scheme. If the inquiry confirms the formal representations, then the properties are closed and demolished.

The community has a duty to rehouse all the inhabitants who were in residence at the time the area was so declared and determined.

Those who take up occupation after this date are not entitled to rehousing for the very good reason that they would gain an unjustified priority of housing by entering a known condemned house, the demolition of which would lead to the offer of immediate accommodation.

Housing and Public Health

Housing standards must meet health requirements. These standards must be enforced if they are to be effective. The responsibility is twofold, firstly that of the architects and builders to see that their work complies with the regulations, and secondly that of the community to carry out inspections and require remedies to be applied where necessary.

Existing houses become obsolete as standards rise; they also wear out with age. They are also liable to be affected indirectly by other building works.

There are provisions for securing the repair, maintenance and sanitary conditions of houses. These are the conditions of:

1. Repair.
2. Stability.
3. Freedom from damp.
4. Natural lighting.
5. Ventilation.
6. Water supply.
7. Drainage and sanitary conveniences.
8. Facilities for storage, preparation and cooking of food and for the disposal of waste water.

The house is considered unfit for human habitation if one or more of the above matters are really defective.

Conditions of letting can be established for people who let small houses. They require the landlord, on letting the house, to put it into a condition reasonably fit for human habitation and to maintain it in that condition.

When a community is satisfied that any house is unfit for human habitation, but can be rendered fit at reasonable cost, they can require the owner by notice to repair the premises. The same compulsion can be applied to a hut, tent, caravan or other temporary or movable shelter, provided it has been in the same place for a reasonable period of time. If the owner does not do the work then the community can do the repairs in his place and claim the cost either in a lump sum or by instalments.

If an owner is unwilling to repair a house which is unfit for human habitation and which cannot be rendered fit at reasonable expense or if the premises are used in contravention of an undertaking not to use them for human habitation, then it should be the duty of the community to make a demolition or closing order or to purchase the house. Such houses if they are officially noted as of architectural or historic interest are not to be demolished, but are closed for human habitation.

The community may make a closing order on any unfit part of a building which is used, or is suitable for use, as a dwelling, or on any underground room which is deemed to be unfit for human habitation.

Standards are required pertaining to rooms where the floor is below the surface of the ground; in the same manner also houses let in lodgings or multiple occupation.

Reference has been made to the demolition of slum property; however, the community has also a responsibility to abate the overcrowding of houses. A dwelling house is considered to be overcrowded at any time when the number of people sleeping in the house is such that two people of opposite sexes and over the age of ten, not being man and wife, must sleep in the same room, or more persons occupy the house than are permitted for the number of rooms and their floor area. In calculating the figure no account is taken of children under one year; those under ten count as half.

The permitted number of people in a dwelling house is the lesser of two figures reckoned as follows, no account being taken of any room having a floor area of less than fifty square feet. It should be noted that the whole house is taken into account and not only the bedrooms.

Overcrowding Table 1

Where a house consists of:

   (a) 1 room   ...   ... 2 persons

(b) 2 rooms ... ... 3 persons
(c) 3 rooms ... ... 5 persons
(d) 4 rooms ... ... 7½ persons
(e) 5 rooms or more ... 10 with an additional 2 for each room in excess of 5.

Overcrowding Table 1
Where the floor area is:

(a) More than 110 square feet 2 persons
(b) 90 to 110 square feet ... 1½ persons
(c) 70 to 90 square feet ... 1 person
(d) 50 to 70 square feet ... ½
(e) Under 50 square feet ... Nil

The landlord should be liable to a penalty for permitting over-crowding. The same applies to the mathematical overcrowding which is caused when a baby attains the age of one or a child passes its tenth birthday.

The community can provide housing accommodation
(a) By erecting houses.
(b) By the conversion of buildings into houses.
(c) By acquiring houses.
(d) By altering, enlarging, repairing or improving houses and buildings.

The community should have powers to fit out, furnish and supply any of their houses with all requisite furniture, fittings and con-veniences and may sell, or supply on a hire purchase agreement, furniture to the occupants of the house.

The community in the first instance must provide houses in order to rehouse tenants from slum clearance and development projects, those suffering from physical and mental ill health, and others in need with urgent social problems.

The demand in many parts of the world for this type of housing has not yet been met. The community has the unenviable task of deciding which of an excessive number of applicants merit the allocation of a house when all are in evident need. If such com-munity housing has been established for several decades, attention must be paid to older couples with grown-up families where under-occupancy exists.

A comprehensive range in size and design of properties is required to meet the changing pattern of a family's evolution. A young newly married couple in theory need a one-bedroom flat. As their children are born larger accommodation, preferably with a garden, is required. The children marry and may stay with their parents for a time, but eventually the needs of the parents revert to one-bedroom accommodation. If and when death severs the partnership, a bed-sittingroom for the surviving partner, with a few treasured possessions, could meet the need.

The development of community housing is often on an estate basis, so that there is multiple construction of one or a few designs suitable for working into a large-scale layout project. This is necessary for ease and speed of construction and also for economy. Under the pressure of scarcity of land and the desire not to scatter dwellings too widely, the modern tendency in towns is to build very tall blocks of municipal flats. These represent a new way of life and set new problems of social and community life to many people whose tradition has been to live in small cottages, or shacks. In addition to the social problems of a concentrated vertical community, many public health problems arise, including the effects of wind and temperature, heating, sewage and refuse disposal, sound-proofing, fire precautions and access for the ambulance service to transport patients.

There is no universal standard for admission to the housing waiting list, or for determining priority. While the intricacies of housing finance and rents are not within the scope of this essay, the transfer of individuals from low rented substandard or slum property to accommodation of higher standard and higher rent, has a bearing on health. The ratio of family income spent on food lessens and impaired health can supervene.

In the priorities, poor health has its place and medical support for a housing application is often forthcoming from an individual's personal medical attendant. The assessment presents three facets, namely the resolution of the personal medical attendant in making a proper and valid judgement, the real need and importunity of the family seeking accommodation, and the needs of others. The community health adviser translates the advice of his medical colleagues to the community housing service.

Community housing sets its own problems. The housing estate forms an artificial group of strangers of roughly the same social class. There are few natural community amenities and no acknowledged community leaders. For the first time in the tenant's lives they are removed from a way of life conditioned by close neighbourliness and often by a family way of life tied to, if not dominated by, the older women of the family. On the one hand there is the stimulus of a new house; on the other there are not the same links with the people next door or across the street; there are heavier expenses in keeping house and goods and transport may cost more. Life is at once easier and more exacting and the full socio-medical effects have yet to be observed of higher material standards, of restricted community activity amounting even to social isolation, and of the opportunity for children and young people to grow up with the support of community medical and educational amenities, though often not supplemented by full social activities.

Plumbing

Plumbing is required in a house to bring in fresh water, to supply cold and hot water within the dwelling to serve radiators, to provide waterborne sanitation and to remove waste.

Water comes from the *service* main through the *service* pipe to the house. An outside *stopcock* is provided to control all the water supply in the communicating pipe from the service mains to the supply pipe on the premises. For convenient control inside the house a *cock* or tap is fitted to the supply pipe. This permits an immediate shut down if there is a minor plumbing mishap inside the house.

The supply pipe leads direct to the cold water taps of the house, the gravity tank of the hot water system and the cistern of the water closets. The cold water connexion is made direct to the '*cold*' taps of baths, sinks, washbasins and any special taps such as garden hose supply points.

The hot water system consists of a means of supply, a method of heating and the necessary supply pipework. A raised gravity supply tank leads into a hot water storage tank. From this hot water is supplied throughout the house by displacement. When a hot water tap is turned on the water in the gravity tank exerts pressure, hot water escapes from the opened tap and the water displaced from the storage tank is replenished by the gravity flow from the high gravity tank. The gravity tank refills by the release of the ball-valve which controls the inlet of cold water from the main.

The water in the storage tank is heated either by circulation from a boiler or by a thermostatically controlled electric or gas heater

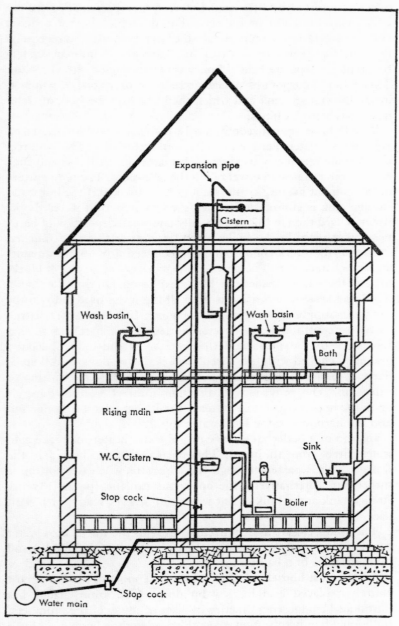

Domestic hot and cold water system.

which is inserted into the actual storage tank. Circulation from a boiler may be direct or indirect. The difference is that a direct system constantly circulates all the water in the storage tank through the boiler by convection, whereas an indirect system re-circulates separate heated boiler water through a closed circuit. This latter incorporates a heat exchanger or *calorifier* which is inside the storage tank and which then heats up the bulk of water in contact with its pipes.

The indirect system continuously re-circulates the same small volume of water between boiler and calorifier. This indirect circulation system can also include radiators in the house and such extra items as a heated towel rail in the bathroom. The temperature in the indirect heating ciruit is not greatly affected if the hot water storage tank is run off and replenished by new cold water. If the water is hard then in this system only one small deposition of hardness takes place in the boiler circuit and after this thin film has formed on the interior of the boiler, the connecting pipes and radiators are not again coated. The bores of the pipes are in no risk of blocking and there is no chance of a boiler explosion. On the other hand, if a direct system of heating is used all the water used daily in the hot water supply passes through the boiler. In a hard water district there are continuing and successive deposits of hardness so that the bores of the pipes and the interior of the boiler becomes gradually choked with fur. Circulation is slowed down and there is likely to be local overheating in the boiler leading to cracking or explosion. The provision of direct or indirect heating depends upon the need to operate a system of radiators from the boiler and also the hardness of the local water supply.

Instead of a boiler an electric or gas water heater may take cold water direct from the main. This normally has to heat only the water which is passed through the apparatus when the hot tap is turned on. Alternatively, the apparatus can incorporate a water storage tank and a bulk of hot water can be kept ready for instant use.

The water closets are connected direct to the mains cold water supply. The supply to replenish the system is provided on demand by the release of a ball valve.

Today most household water pipes are copper. This has almost entirely replaced lead in new buildings. The same change has introduced engineering practice in place of much of the plumbers' traditional handicraft. Nowadays this leadwork is largely confined to repairs. For some work galvanized steel pipe is used as an alternative to copper: in recent years polythene piping has been tried.

In addition to the cold and hot water systems, waste water disposal, water closet waste connections and rain water pipes have to be provided.

Waste water is disposed of by a waste pipe with a *trap* so designed as to seal off the return flow of air by this route. The trap is inside the building and is to be found immediately under the sink, washbasin or bath which it serves.

The traditional, effective but inelegant S-trap is now being replaced in positions where it is conspicuous by other more attractive designs. These still embody the same principle of using some of the waste water in a pocket to seal off any return flow of air and also provide a means of removing foreign matter from a sump at the base.

Venting through the waste pipe is of little public health significance but such traps stop the distasteful ingress of odour and also the entry of a variety of insects and other small game.

The waste pipe must discharge into the drain over a trapped gully. This is the familiar device at ground level, covered by a ribbed or perforated metal grid with a sump beneath which can be cleansed of any precipitated matter. The reason for the demand for a ventilated trap is to stop a direct connexion between waste pipe and drain so that the foul air from the drain cannot enter the house by means of the waste. A century ago 'sewer gas' was considered a major cause of infectious disease. This view is now known to be wrong; but methane and hydrogen sulphide are unpleasant and if not checked could occur in a sufficient concentration to be debilitating quite apart from their effects both aesthetic and in terms of mental ill health.

Water closets vary in the detail of their design. The modern device is a one-piece seat pedestal with a rim designed to aid flushing. The base is formed over an S-trap to prevent the back flow of foul air. The closet usually has a lifting seat and a flap lid though these may be replaced by some simple seating where there is much public resort and a risk of fouling. The water-closet is connected to the drain by a vented wastepipe. This means merely that at a convenient level the waste passes into a vertical cast-iron pipe, usually four inches in diameter. The upper end projects six feet above the highest window. The open upper end acts as a vent to the drain and relieves any pressure changes in the system when in use. This protects the closet water seals from displacement by pressure when another water-closet is flushed. Rats may enter the drains and climb inside the vertical vent pipes. To stop their escape out of the top, the upper opening of each vent is fitted with a spherical wire basket which acts as an impassable barrier to rats. It also stops birds from plugging the opening by nest building.

Rainwater is collected from roofs by horizontal gutters slightly inclined so that the water runs freely to *downpipes*. These discharge over a trapped gully into a drain; in districts where underground wells are used for the public water supply the rainwater is often passed into soakways which permit it to percolate down through porous strata to add to the well contents. Where rainwater is drained away it may be disposed of on the *combined system* through the general sewers or, more efficiently, it may be led away through separate storm-water sewers.

The connexions for waste water, closet discharge and also rainwater where the combined system is used is by underground drains. These pipes are laid in a straight line with a slight declivity or *fall*. They meet in brick or concrete *inspection chambers*. These are junction boxes where the channels are open and solid refuse can be removed or rods can be introduced for clearing obstructions in the various drains entering the chamber. The inspection chambers have an airtight metal lid to seal off the contents from the external air.

13
Food and Health

To survive, man needs respirable air, a sufficiency of drinking water and food and and a climate in which he can survive with the means available to him.

The water balance of a sedentary man is based on a daily intake and output of some two and a half litres of which one and a half litres are drunk and excreted as urine while the other litre is ingested in food or created inside the body by oxygenation and is lost by the water content or the expired air of respiration, by perspiration and by moisture in the faeces. This water balance has to be adjusted to exertion and to the control of body temperature with consequent variations in intake offset by perspiration and respiration.

Any fresh water will meet the physical needs of the body but if the water is contaminated there is at once a hazard to health.

Food must be adequate in quantity and contain a sufficient amount of all these substances which are necessary for the physiological demands of the body for energy and for the maintenance and replacement of tissue.

The average man needs about 3,000 calories in the daily diet assuming that 10 per cent will be lost due to incomplete digestion and absorption.

The heat values of protein, fat and carbohydrate are set out below:

1 g Protein	...	...	...	4 calories
1 g Fat	...	...	...	9 calories
1 g Carbohydrate	...	...	...	4 calories

A man doing moderate muscular work needs the following diet:

Protein	100 g	...	...	400 calories
Fat	100 g	...	...	900 calories
Carbohydrate	500 g	...	...	2,000 calories
				3,300 calories

An average woman requires about 80 per cent of a man's needs with adjustment according to occupation.

The diet, in addition to being adequate in its major items, must contain the appropriate vitamins and trace metals. The food must be of a consistency to promote dental hygiene by chewing and the rapid onward removal of carbohydrates so potentially harmful to the teeth. The food must be digestible and contain a sufficient quantity of indigestible material to form an adequate bulk and consistency of faeces and so to promote proper defaecation.

Man is an active human being on whom civilization has imposed a largely sedentary way of life. This has become aggravated in Europe in the present century by the improvement and spread of public transport so that walking and other unavoidable exercise has been reduced to a minimum.

Studies have shown that those having occupations involving continuous and vigorous exercise have a lower tendency to cardio-vascular degeneration. If such exercise cannot be achieved in the daily occupation then its equivalent must be obtained by deliberately seeking some form of recreational exercise. It is better to provide this by reasonable daily walking or gardening than by attempting brief episodes of violent exertion for which the sedentary body has lost or never has had adequate training.

Milk

The production of milk is an organized rural industry with all the problems involved in management, staffing, the environment and the product itself.

Milk which is an ideal food is at the same time a potentially harmful substance, by reason of its ideal composition as a medium for the growth of pathogenic bacteria. Unhygienic production, transport, processing and distribution can all contribute to its pollution.

Milk is now collected in bulk and delivered to dairy factories for processing, bottling and delivery. Only a small proportion is bottled on the farm and distributed direct.

As a culture medium milk can be infected by systemic infection from the cow (tuberculosis, brucellosis and, rarely, anthrax and foot-and-mouth disease). The cow's udder may be secondarily infected from a carrier (*streptococci*, *B. diphtherae*). There may be breaches in food hygiene permitting access of infection from without

(typhoid, paratyphoid) either by the presence of a carrier or by
the use of infected water either for washing utensils or fraudulently
to dilute the milk. A variety of organisms will grow on neglected or
ill-washed equipment if the film of old milk is not removed. This
at once introduces a personal factor with regard to the standards to be
maintained by the labour force in handling the milk and equipment.

The two alternative methods of producing and handling milk are
to rely on 'safe' milk from tuberculosis-free herds and to distribute
it rapidly before it deteriorates or to rely on heat treatment to
pasteurize the milk and so make it bacteriologically safe.

There are few topics more the field of the controversialist than
that of food: milk has not escaped. Suffice it to say that any policy
of selling raw milk from tuberculosis-free animals can leave the
way wide open for every milk-borne disease except tuberculosis
itself. Pasteurization renders milk safe by the elimination of pathogenic bacteria and so eliminates not only tuberculosis but all other
hazards.

Bovine tuberculosis is a disappearing disease due to the combined effects of compulsory heat treatment of milk and the sub-
sidies which in a generation have substituted tuberculosis-free
dairy herds for a situation where the milk of cattle showing a
national average of forty per cent tuberculosis infection was
retailed raw for human consumption.

In the United Kingdom there are four special designations of
milk—untreated, pasteurized, sterilized and ultra heat treated—
and tests for standard have been laid down. Producers and dealers
are licensed and the licensing conditions enable control to be
exercised at every point during the production, handling, heat
treatment, storage and distribution of milk. An administrative
technique is the declaration of 'specified areas' in which only the
specially designated milk may be sold. Thus quite strict control is
exercised over milk supplies and a high proportion of such supplies
are heat treated.

In the United Kingdom a high proportion of the country's milk
supplies comes from tuberculin-tested cattle. However, a programme of total heat treated milk is essential to prevent the transmission of *Brucella abortus* in milk from infected beasts to humans.

Standards are imposed on the design and conduct of byres and
milking parlours. Milk is filtered at once then cooled to 10°C. It
should be kept covered at all times to prevent access to dust. Milk
may be bottled on the farm with or without prior pasteurization.

More usually it is transported by road or rail in either churns or tanks to a central processing plant where it is pasteurized, bottled and distributed for delivery to the consumer.

The classical process for pasteurization is the 'Holder process' whereby milk is retained at a temperature of 62·8°–65·6°C. for at least half an hour and then immediately cooled to 10°C. The alternative, which is almost universal, is the High Temperature Short Time (HTST) process whereby the milk is held at a temperature of not less than 71·7°C for at least fifteen seconds and immediately cooled to 10°C. There are variants of the process but essentially the same procedures are adopted.

Sterilization may be used instead of pasteurization. The heating to 100°C for one hour permits the milk to keep well but reduces its nutritional value and changes its flavour. Sterilized milk is hygienically safe: it is attractive to housewives as it is remixed by homogenization so that the cream is evenly distributed through the bulk. This gives a creamier taste.

Dried milk is prepared by being sprayed on the surface of rotating metal cylinders, heated to 140°C. The thin film of milk dries on the surface and is carried past knife-edged scrapers which remove it in flakes. It is then pulverized and packed. Another method is to force the previously pasteurized milk in a fine spray into a chamber containing air at 115°C. The milk dries to powder in the air and falls to the bottom of the chamber whence it is removed for packing.

Dried milk packed in air-tight tins keeps well especially if gas-packed so that it is stored in an atmosphere of nitrogen which protects the remaining 80 per cent of Vitamin C. Dried milk represents a concentration of seven or eight times that of normal milk.

In the United Kingdom Dried Milk legal standards are as below:

Description of Dried Milk	% Milk Fat
Dried full cream Milk	Not less than 26
,, ¾ ,, ,,	Less than 26 more than 17
,, ½ ,, ,,	Not more than 17 not less than 14
,, ¼ ,, ,,	Less than 14 and not less than 8
,, Partly skimmed Milk	Less than 8 and not less than 1·5
,, Skimmed Milk	Less than 1·5

Partly skimmed dried milk (containing between 8 per cent and 1·5 per cent of milk fat) should not be used for babies except under medical advice and skimmed dried milk (with less than 1·5 per cent milk fat) is unfit for babies.

Condensed Milk

The concentration of condensed milk is three times that of normal milk.

The unsweetened variety is packed in tins and sterilized in pressure cookers at 115°C. Sweetened milk is concentrated with sugar and is not sterile, though it is pasteurized at the beginning of processing.

There are six types of condensed milk: full cream (sweetened and unsweetened), half cream (sweetened and unsweetened) and skimmed (sweetened and unsweetened).

Half cream condensed milk must be labelled as 'Not to be used for babies except under medical advice' and the skimmed variety has to bear a categorical statement that it is 'unfit for babies.'

Sterilized milk is packed in bottles sealed with crown corks.

Milk Bottle Washing

Dirty bottles can spoil efficiently pasteurized milk.

Modern bottle washing machines provide soaking and rinsing with clean hot water and the use of soda or detergents. After this the bottles are virtually sterile. They should be stored upside down if they cannot be refilled at once. To prevent soiling of the bottle neck modern bottle caps cover the whole of the rim of the neck. The original internal diaphragm bottle seal of cardboard was itself a great advance but it is now obsolete. The use of disposable cartons is excellent but expensive in a country that has no native wood-pulp industry. Plastic bottles have been suggested, and offer a further advantage in the reduction of the early morning noise nuisance from delivery vehicles.

Meat

Sound meat in good condition is a most valuable part of a mixed diet. It is essential that food animals be healthy before slaughter, the abattoir and its conduct be hygienic and the storage, transport and disposal of the meat be carried out to the strict standards of a code of practice, including a legal one. All carcases must be inspected for disease at the time of slaughter and dressing.

If the following signs and symptoms are detected then an animal should not be received into the main abattoir where meat is slaughtered for human consumption: Shivers, hot muzzle, hanging head, dull eyes, rough coat, nasal discharge, cough, rapid breathing, watery dung with blood or mucus; loss of appetite, distended abdomen, oedema, septic wounds or skin conditions. The normal pulse for a beast is 40: the normal rectal temperature is 101·5°F (38·4°C).

Special isolation provision should be made for sick or injured animals.

Some special diseases of animals must be identified whenever possible.

Their main features are set out below:

Anthrax

Generally ill, blood in stools and urine, fever with increased pulse. The diagnosis is made by the demonstration of anthrax bacilli in a sample of blood taken from the ear. This is a hazardous procedure which should be left to the veterinarian or bacteriologist.

Foot-and-Mouth Disease

Vesicles on feet, mouth, tongue and udder; nasal discharge; fever.

Tuberculosis

In cattle and pigs, rarely sheep or goats.

Cough, rapid respiration, emaciation, nodules in udder. Positive tuberculin reaction.

Pleuro-pneumonia

Generally ill, dyspnoea, tenderness on pressure over ribs, symptoms of pneumonia.

Unfit Meat

Meat may be unfit for consumption by reason of illness in the animal prior to slaughter: the animal may be exposed to infection in the last few days of life and the condition may show itself only in the lairs or even post-mortem.

In particular bottle-fed calves of a few days old, especially in transit, are liable to bowel infections which can be transmitted to humans. The practice of slaughtering these very young animals is not sound on health grounds. An older, heavy calf of three months or more is a much better product all round.

The carcase may be contaminated during the process of dressing after slaughter; by unhygienic handling and storage it can be soiled or damaged at any stage from the abattoir to the moment of retail sale.

Slaughterhouses

The community must be responsible for the control of the hygiene of slaughterhouses. The essentials for a slaughterhouse are an adequate water supply and a system of sewage disposal able to cope with the repeated washing down and removal of general filth from roadways and lairs as well as the post-mortem refuse associated with slaughtering and dressing. The buildings must include lairs, slaughter halls fitted with shooting pens, hanging rooms for the carcases to cool off, cold storage, offal and hide stores, a condemned meat room, destructor and manure dump as well as a boiler house, offices, sanitary accommodation, and dressing and changing rooms for the slaughtermen and the administrative staff. As by-products will be involved, facilities should be provided on the spot for tripe boiling and dressing, gut scraping, blood boiling, bone processing and the like.

All animals must be inspected as soon as possible after slaughter. The normal procedure is set out below.

Head

Examine the jaw for actinomycosis, the lips, tongue and nostrils for foot-and-mouth disease and the submaxillary, retropharyngeal and parotid glands for tuberculosis. In addition, the masseters are repeatedly incised to examine for the presence of *Cysticercus bovis*.

Tongue

Examine for actinobacillosis (woody tongue), and *Cysticercus bovis*.

Lungs

Tuberculosis, parasitic cysts, pneumonia.
Examine bronchial and mediastinal glands.

Heart

Incise for *Cysticercus bovis*.

K

Liver

Tuberculosis, abscesses, necrosis, parasites. Examine hepatic glands.

Stomach

Examine peritoneal surface and glands for tuberculosis.

Spleen

Anthrax, tuberculosis.

Mesentery

Examine glands.

Udder

Tubercular abscesses or mastitis. Examine glands.

Carcase examination

Haemorrhage, emaciation, oedema, emphysema, bruising or jaundice. Sight parietal pleura and peritoneum (which should never be removed; if this is missing the carcase should be rejected). There should be no unpleasant odour.

Meat in good condition is a lively light red with the fat just off white. It should be firm and moist. Decomposition alters this appearance.

The head and tail, lungs, heart, liver, spleen, kidneys, pancreas and tongue are commercially known as offal.

The main reasons for meat being condemned as unfit are as follows:

Tuberculosis. Differential diagnosis—pyaemic abscesses especially in liver, lungs, kidney and spleen; cysticercosis and echinococcus cysts; caseous lymphadenitis and actinomycosis.

Caseous lymphadenitis occurs mainly in sheep. It is the practice to condemn the quarter of the animal in which it is detected.

Actinomycosis affects the tongue, jaws and occasionally the lungs. Usually only the affected region of the carcase is condemned.

Anthrax, pyaemia and septicaemia require the destruction of the carcase. In anthrax the carcase is burnt or buried in lime.

Among other conditions demanding the condemnation of the carcase are erysipelas, foot-and-mouth disease, jaundice, septic conditions, multiple swellings or tumours in muscles, and swine fever.

Infestation by parasites must be looked for. *Taenia saginata* in its cysticercal form occurs in cattle as minute pearly cysts usually in the muscle of the head, neck, shoulders, heart. It is most conveniently sought by a dozen parallel cuts into the masseter muscle. The carcase can be condemned or, if the cysts are thought to be non-viable by reason of surrounding calcification, the carcase can be refrigerated for three weeks and then used for 'industrial' purposes involving bulk cooking.

Taenia solium may be detected in pigs as *Cysticercus* cellulosae. If infestation is found the carcase should be condemned.

Trichinella spiralis occurs in pigs in the *cysticercus* stage. The cysts are invisible unless calcified when they are seen on the muscles as tiny white specks especially around the tendon insertions.

Slaughter of animals

After shooting through the forehead with the humane killer, which is a pistol with a captive bolt projectile, cattle are 'pithed' with a cane, hung up, bled and the hide flayed off. The carcase is opened and the offal and head are set aside for inspection. The carcase is split in two through the midline and after inspection the two halves are hung in a cool airy room for the temperature gradually to fall. After twelve hours the carcase is fit for onward disposal usually into a chill-room for temporary storage and conditioning. Attempts to speed up matters by artificial cooling are likely to lead to bone-taint which is a form of putrefaction of the deeper muscles.

Sheep, calves and lambs are shot in the same way as cattle; pigs may be shot but it is convenient to stun them with an electro-lethaler. This is an insulated device rather like a big pair of coal tongs carrying saline soaked pads at its extremities. The pads are applied to both temples of the pig. The pressure of contact switches on an electric current in the pads and so stuns the pig. The animal is hung up, its carotid arteries opened to bleed it, the hairs are removed from the skin either by hand, by flaming or mechanically and the carcase is dressed and hung to cool before going to cold store.

The practice of importing live cattle into a country must be positively discouraged and be replaced by the importation of dressed carcase meat preserved either by freezing at — 7°C or chilling at — 2° to — 1°C. Chilled meat will keep for about three weeks but frozen meat will keep for two or three years. The essential difference is the damaging effect of the lower temperature on the tissues: frozen meat is less attractive though equally nutritious. Meat should be transported and distributed in special vans with a smooth, easily cleaned interior. The meat should not be stacked but should be hung from racks; offal and small pieces should be kept in metal dishes or containers. Those carrying the meat should be personally clean and should wear washable overalls and caps.

Fish

The only special problem about fish as a foodstuff is its liability to deterioration. It is edible immediately after being caught: the longer the time interval between catching and consumption, the poorer the condition.

Sea fish caught in distant waters has to be preserved on ice with the addition of antibiotic until it can be landed. It deteriorates rapidly when removed. As fish becomes stale the tissues soften and pit on pressure; the eye, previously clear, sinks and the gills become discoloured. There is a tendency for the skin to loosen and the flesh shrinks away from the bones. The same problem of general hygiene exist as with meat, milk and other protein-containing foods.

New fishing techniques are being allied to processing methods at sea so that the fish is packed and deep-frozen aboard the vessel. This will reduce handling to a minimum. There are no parasites worthy of note except *Diphyllubothrium latum* which is rare in this country. It is transmitted to man by eating raw fish or caviare.

Shellfish

Shellfish are excellent biological filters. By their feeding habits they extract bacteria from the water. In so doing they accumulate the bacteria within their bodies. If uncooked shellfish contaminated by pathogenic bacteria are eaten by man then he will become infected in his turn. The risk is a very real one when the shellfish come from 'laying' sited near sewage outfalls.

The main risk in this country is from typhoid. *B. typhosum* and *V. cholerae* as well as *E. coli* will survive in sea-water for some days. This varies according to climatic and meteorological conditions.

The main shellfish eaten in Britain are cockles, mussels, whelks, winkles and oysters. The standards of permissible bacterial contamination and categories are set out below: *E. coli faecalis* is used as an indicator.

E. coli (Faecal Type I) per ml of Flesh	
	Conclusion
5 colonies	Quite satisfactory.
6–15 colonies	Suspicious. Further samples to be taken. Sale not immediately prohibited.
Above 15 colonies	Unsatisfactory. Sale prohibited until further samples examined.

Due to their method of feeding, shellfish are a reservoir of bacteria, some of which may be harmful. They can be made safe by two different methods of cleansing: either by placing the shellfish in large tanks filled with sterile water which is changed every 24 hours for 2 to 3 days, or by placing them in tanks with a constant supply of water sterilized by ultra-violet light for 36 hours. Because both processes involve the shellfish actively feeding, the salinity and temperature of the water must be maintained.

At certain seasons the gonads of some fish and shellfish can cause toxic effects when eaten. This may be the explanation of associated episodes of food poisoning in which no causative organism can be demonstrated.

Preservation of Foodstuffs

Traditional methods of preserving foodstuffs are by drying, salting and the use of natural cold.

The preservation of figs and dates, the preparation of biltong in South Africa and pemmican in North America, the eating of frozen mammoths recovered from the ice of Siberia, the freezing of sides of beef in the rigging of old-time whalers bound for the Arctic, the ancient preservation of fish and meat by smoking over wood fires or by salting are but a few examples of traditional practice.

Modern methods include refrigeration either by chilling or by freezing, smoking, canning or bottling and exposure to high temperature, dehydration, chemical preservation and gas storage.

Low temperature preservation is applied to animal foods, meat, fish, eggs, milk and dairy produce. 'Deep freezing' at below zero temperatures is used for all foodstuffs.

Smoking is confined to bacon, ham and herrings. Oak or other hard wood is used in the smoking-houses.

Canning and bottling make use of the principle of pasteurization, tyndallization or cooking in order to destroy organisms and spores. After packing and heating, bottles are sealed: tins are sealed before heating. Cans may be defective by reason of leaks, strain due to over-packing, under sterilization, blowing due to the generation of gas or collapse due to too high a final vacuum associated with underfilling.

The 'blowing' of tins can be due to the generation of putrefactive gases or by harmless 'hydrogen swell' due to the acid contents especially of fruit or vegetables acting on the iron of the can where it is not protected by internal lacquering. In either case the tins and their contents should be rejected as defective. When gas is generated in preserving bottles the vacuum seal is lost, the lids lift and become loose permitting the entry of external air and spores with consquent further deterioration.

Tins are inspected for holes, indentation and general damage. Extensive rust is a risk as it can lead to perforation. The joints may be damaged or there may be 'swell' or 'blowing'. Palpation may give the first indication of fullness due to blowing. Percussion may aid in the detection.

Meat is solid: decomposition should be suspected if the tin is shaken and the contents sound liquid.

Botulism from canned vegetables is so rare in Britain that it may be regarded as a curiosity: lead and tin may be taken up by canned fish in excess of the amounts permitted. The former theory of 'ptomaine poisoning' from deteriorated canned meat and similar foods is now known to be a fallacy: for food to putrefy to an extent where ptomaines form means that at the same time it would be too unpalatable to eat. The risk to opened cans of food is the same as to other food, namely the hazards of external bacteria flourishing if kept at room temperature instead of in a refrigerator.

Preservation of food by drying depends upon the removal of the moisture necessary for bacterial growth. Drying can be natural, in the sun, or by artificial heat. The mean water content is 2% but some foods dry at 5% and others at 0·5%. Some foods may be reconstituted with water before consumption. Fruit, vegetables, milk, eggs, meat and fish can be preserved in this way.

Modern methods permit the drying of vegetables while preserving their colour. Dried vegetables prepared by modern methods keep a great part of their vitamin content. They also keep well in storage.

Eggs are spray dried, they reconstitute at the rate of 10 eggs to a pound of liquid. Meat drying is difficult as the process which is successful with minced meat is not adequate for bigger pieces.

In dehydrating food the water content must be reduced, the enzymes must be destroyed by short heat treatment before drying, oxygen must be excluded when possible; the water content of the dried product must be kept low during storage; the drying must be at not too high a temperature though drying itself must be rapid, the material while still moist must be kept at a temperature other than that at which bacteria flourish.

All this is of little use if the best materials are not provided. Full food hygiene methods must always be carried out.

The exclusion of air as a method of preservation has long been known. Home potted meat is preserved by an upper layer of butter or margarine melted and allowed to set.

Eggs may be greased or stored in a solution of waterglass (sodium tri-silicate).

Modern scientific methods control the temperature, humidity and gas content of the storage atmosphere. This is applied to fruit, meat, bacon and eggs.

Food which is stored for a long time in ordinary containers is liable to become infested by insects, mites and other parasites.

Sometimes foodstuffs arriving from abroad are already infested.

Others become infested by being place in contact with other material, by being packed in sacks or boxes or by being stored in an infested store-room. Even a brief period in a transport vehicle may be sufficient to pass on the infestation.

There are a large variety of infesting insects often limited to one foodstuff.

Tyroglyphus farinae:	flour mite.
Tyrolichus casei:	cheese mite.
Tyrophagus castellani:	copra itch mite.

Pediculoides ventricosus:	grain itch mite.
Carpoglyphus lactis:	dried fruit mite.
Ephestia kuhniella:	mill moth (flour, cereals).
Ephestia elutella:	cacao moth.
Ephestia cautella:	fig moth.
Plodia interpunctella:	Indian meal moth.
Endrosis saratrella:	pulses, cereals.
Calandra granaria:	grain weevil.
Calandra oryzea:	rice weevil.
Stegobium paniceum:	bread beetle.
Ptinus tectus:	brown spider beetle.

In addition, certain insects foul food or carry dirt and infection. These include cockroaches (*Blatta orientalis*) and steam flies (*Blatella germanica*) as well as Pharaoh's ant (*Monomonium pharaonis*).

The *prevention and control of infestation* depends upon the original foodstuff being free from infestation, being stored in pest-free containers and rooms and being protected against infestation. Food stores should be cool and airy and not provide harbourage for pests. This is achieved by seeing that there are no cracks or crevices which can form refuges or nests: accumulations of old food and of rubbish which can form retreats should not be permitted. This requires a model standard of cleanliness. Regular inspection is necessary and any signs of infestation should at once be rooted out. Incoming stock should be sighted. If possible metal bins should be used. In bulk storage this is impossible. The stock must be divided and stacked in sections with gangways to minimize a widespread infestation.

The community has a role and a responsibility to ensure that food is produced, processed, and distributed within standards to eradicate any potential hazard to the consumer. Food can be injurious to health by nature of its quality, constitution or potency due to the addition or abstraction of any substance. A cumulative effect of harmful substances must be borne in mind.

If the nature, substance, or quality of any food distributed for human consumption is not of the standard demanded, then an offence has been committed. Governments have powers to regulate and control additives to food, some of which may be accidental such as pesticide residues. Any decision to use, or not to use, a particular chemical in food or in the environment has to be carefully related to many factors, including sociological or ecological ones, obtaining in the locality in which the chemical is to be used.

Health officers within a community have powers to sample food for submission to a public analyst. The substances can be taken at the time of preparation, and at any point of distribution and sale.

With the advent of bulk containerization, the sampling of the food at the point where the containers are broken down is of obvious importance. Powers exist for health officers on warrant to enter premises, if need be by force, if there are reasonable grounds for entry, even, in a matter of urgency, if the premises are unoccupied. Any food intended for human consumption can be examined at any reasonable time and if it appears unfit, it may be seized. If a justice confirms its unsoundness, then the food is condemned and destroyed.

Animal meat or meat products from a knacker's yard may not be sold for human consumption.

Society can make regulations about food hygiene in connexion with the sale, importation, preparation, transport, storage, packaging, wrapping, exposure for sale, service or delivery of food for human consumption.

Requirements can be laid down for:

(a) The construction, layout, drainage, equipment, maintenance, cleanliness, ventilation, lighting, water supply and use of premises in or from which food is sold for human consumption, including parts where utensils are cleaned and also that part where refuse is stored or disposed of.

(b) The provision and maintenance of sanitary and washing facilities, the disposal of refuse and the maintenance and cleanliness of apparatus, equipment, furnishings and utensils and particularly the supply of flushing water to every sanitary convenience.

(c) The prohibition or control of special materials in making food-handling equipment.

(d) The prohibition of smoking on food premises.

(e) Specifying details of clothing of food handlers.

(f) The inspection of animals, including poultry, for slaughter, and their carcases and meat.

(g) The staining or sterilization of unfit meat.

(h) The disposal of unfit food.

(i) The prohibition or control of the sale of shellfish.

Codes of good catering and food hygiene practice can be published for the advice and guidance of all concerned.

It is considered by some authorities that all food premises should be registered. Others take the more restricted view about the sale, manufacture or storage of ice-cream, or the preparation and manufacture of sausages, or potted, pressed, pickled or preserved food.

Such registration can be cancelled if the requirements or standards are not met. Vehicles, stalls, and places to be used for food premises should also be registered.

Special measures are required to prevent the spread of disease by ice-cream. Every manufacturer or dealer should notify the community health officer of the occurrence of disease among his staff.

Any ice-cream or ingredients if suspected may be immobilized, and on confirmation of suspicion must be destroyed.

Special attention must be paid to sale of horse-flesh and the cleansing of shellfish.

As previously indicated, milk from the farm, dairy, and its manufactured products (cream, butter, cheese, dried and condensed milk) are candidates for particularly detailed regulations. There should be prohibition of the sale of milk from diseased cows with such clinical entities as acute mastitis, actinomycosis of udder, suppuration of udder, infection of udder, any comatose condition, any septic condition of uterus, anthrax and foot-and-mouth disease. It is an offence to adulterate milk.

The community may establish and acquire markets with definition of market days and hours.

Slaughterhouses and knackers' yards have to be licensed. Cold stores and refrigerators may be provided by the community.

REFERENCE

The British Nutrition Foundation Ltd. *Information Bulletin* (1970) No. 4, p. 16.

14

Occupational Health

OCCUPATIONAL health goes far beyond the narrower field of health in industry: if the term is logically applied it includes the health of schoolchildren, housewives and other significant groups. Occupational health services deal effectively with the problems of fishermen and seamen, agricultural workers, transport workers and others whose working life is spent outside the factory or mine.

The health and safety of workpeople is affected by a large variety of factors.

Legal requirements demand attention to safety, hygiene, deleterious conditions and the prevention of accidents and industrial diseases.

Other safeguards include the following:

(i) Study of toxic hazards.
(ii) The use of harmless substances in place of those which are toxic.
(iii) Limitation of exposure.
(iv) Prevention of dust and fumes.
(v) Protective apparatus.
(vi) Cleanliness of work-places.
(vii) General hygiene.
(viii) Prohibition of long hours especially for females and young people.
(ix) Bodily cleanliness.
(x) Medical inspection on entry and at intervals.
(xi) Selection of workpeople.
(xii) Replacement of manual labour by mechanical aids.

Industrial health has a longer official history in Britain than has public health. The main advances, apart from the reduction and final abolition of child labour, have been in the reduction of working hours, improvements in safety and the elimination of toxic hazards.

From the beginning of the Industrial Revolution pauper children were hired to contractors to work in coal-mines, cotton and woollen mills and on the land.

Then legislation was introduced to control the working hours of children and women later extended to the guarding of machinery and dust control.

It has long been known that adverse working conditions cause ill health. History records extreme episodes of this in the fate of Mediterranean galley slaves and of conscript miners in the gold-mines of Spanish South America.

In 1780 a Swedish minister of religion noted the ravages of silicosis among cutlers: in his words 'all live to twenty, some to thirty but none survive till forty'.

Brassfounders' ague, chimney-sweeps' cancer, miners' phthisis, bakers' itch are names attached to specific industrial conditions: their familiar designation reveals their former frequency.

Many of these conditions are preventable and most can be held in check by proper thought and preventive action. Though preventive industrial medicine and especially toxicology is a fascinating subject the vast majority of hazards can be eliminated from work when there is proper attention to cleanliness, accident prevention and ventilation.

There are a large number of specific industrial hazards. Since these have been recognized their effects have been largely nullified. In general throughout industry new processes are now carefully examined and planned from the outset to minimize or eliminate risk. This awareness means that accident or carelessness involving relatively common chemicals in any of a large number of processes are the real risk and not, as in former days, the results of some single special process involving an unrecognized but dangerous component.

Nine-tenths of industrial ill health is due to sepsis following trauma: rheumatism causes the greater part of the remainder: only a small proportion of all morbidity results from specific toxic hazards.

Sepsis is reduced by proper attention to personal cleanliness both on the job and at home. Dirty working clothes hold general dirt and sometimes specifically harmful substances in contact with the skin so that frequent provision of clean overalls and clothing is essential both for hygiene and for protection. A clean place of work contributes to general hygiene, to the elimination of dust, oil and other potentially harmful substances.

Accident prevention in industry is linked with careful job selection, good management, a self-disciplined, trained and contented labour force, safe working conditions and an active education policy in accident prevention.

Handicapped workpeople can make a useful contribution to industry when properly occupied within their limitations. More than forty years ago Henry Ford in the U.S.A. initiated an employment policy based on using the same proportion of handicapped people as existed in the general community. In his factories a proportion of blind, deaf, crippled, limbless, epileptic and other disabled people were placed in jobs suitable for them.

Handicapped people in the wrong job are a hazard to themselves and to others. The nature and extent of each individual handicap should be studied in relation to the proposed job. What at first sight appears to be a gross disability may not be of any consequence when its effect on the task is carefully analysed.

Some people are accident-prone by reason of personality and mental make-up. Adolescents are specifically forbidden to operate certain categories of machinery which incorporate a hazard for it is held that immaturity may induce an irresponsible attitude to a very real risk.

Good management means a general atmosphere of anticipation of risk and a positive willingness to adjust matters as soon as possible.

Given the best possible working conditions accidents will always happen if the workmen do not take their share in prevention. The first requirement is self-discipline. If the work is only casual then the approach to it is casual: if the work is steady and there is a reasonable guarantee of a job for as long as it is wanted then a tradition of work emerges and a code of practice develops. If introductory training and safety instruction has been given this will be blended into the general attitude towards accident prevention measures and to the educative propaganda which itself ought never to be relaxed and which should be aimed at all grades from management to the workshop floor. Safe working conditions are partly dependent upon the workman and partly on management. Safety devices can be incorporated in machinery and processes but they must not be put out of action for the selfish convenience of the individual. If protective eyeshields, clothing, footgear, gloves and the like are provided they are meant to be used. The securing of ladders and work stages, safe hoisting and lifting, the fitting of guard-rails and toe-boards on scaffoldings and high openings, the closing of manholes and trap-doors, the removal of obstructions which cause tripping and falling are only a few of the individual actions which cause or obviate accidents irrespective of the type of work. Adequate lighting over the job and at awkward places, the cleaning of floors, the provision of white lines for restricting obstruction, attention to wear and tear and defect, especially in electrical apparatus, care in handling acids and other harmful substances, arrangements for workmen leaving the factory without traffic risk are other headings under which accident prevention is achieved.

Health education about accident prevention should start with a careful explanation of the general precautions in the workplace as well as the special precautions necessary on the job itself. The initial industrial training should emphasize the care and attention which is necessary to avoid risk.

The main concern in education is to disperse apathy, stimulate interest and eliminate undesirable procedures. This requires a policy of continuous application of accident prevention propaganda designed above all to be stimulating and to arouse interest. Intermittent, ill-conceived or badly handled attacks on the problem have little impact and may even acclimatize resistance so that good propaganda is ignored.

Specific Industrial Hazards

Carbon dioxide causes simple asphyxia.

It is associated with irrespirable atmospheres in wells, silos, breweries, ships' holds and the cleaning of tanks. If there is more than 10 per cent of carbon dioxide in the air it becomes unfit to support life.

Carbon monoxide is the most common cause of gassing in industry. It is odourless. The gas has a greater affinity for haemoglobin than oxygen and replaces it so that oxygen exchange in the circulation stops. Carbon monoxide in sufficient concentration renders its victims helpless without warning. Rescue is not possible in an atmosphere of carbon monoxide except by the use of breathing apparatus.

Artificial respiration and the use of oxygen with 7 per cent carbon dioxide as a respiratory stimulant is the best treatment even though the blood is defective in its function of oxygenation due to the irreversible affinity of carbon monoxide for the haemoglobin.

Carbon monoxide occurs in motor exhausts, domestic gas,

blast-furnace gases, mine explosions and the operation of coke ovens.

Sulphuretted Hydrogen is associated with the collection and decomposition of organic materials and in processes in the chemical and gas industries. It can be fatal in a concentration of 1 part per 1000.

Sulphur dioxide, chlorine and ammonia are a hazard as leaks from chemical processes. They are irritant to the bronchial tree and produce copious watery secretion with coughing. If the exposure has been sufficient the patient may drown in his own secretions.

Nitrous fumes are brown in colour. They occur when nitric acid is spilt or acts upon metal with the formation of nitric oxide and nitrogen peroxide. They are also a by-product of arc welding and of the detonation or burning of explosives. The risk occurs from their delayed action: there is an initial irritation followed by a period of hours of *well-being* after which there is a sudden onset of pulmonary oedema.

The history is characteristic and on it alone the patient should be placed lying at rest and have oxygen administered continuously.

Any nitrous fumes are a risk unless immediately and efficiently removed: all risk must be got out of the way until the hazard has been dealth with. Escaped nitric acid must be diluted by an overwhelming volume of water and adequate ventilation provided.

Lead poisoning is but rarely acute: the chronic form is more common. *Acute* lead poisoning is characterized by colic, wrist drop, or foot drop. Acute lead encephalopathy or convulsions may be seen. The end result may be blindness, paralysis and insanity.

Lead is stored cumulatively in the body. The resultant chronic lead poisoning is ushered in by malaise and anaemia. The characteristic blue line due to lead sulphide appears at the gum edge particularly in those who neglect the use of the toothbrush. There may be colic. A toxic nephritis occurs with oedema. This is associated with albuminuria and hyperpiesis with a risk of cerebral haemorrhage.

The blood shows punctate basophilia of the erythrocytes. Peripheral neuritis and paralysis may occur. The patient may lose his teeth. In pregnant women abortion is a feature of the syndrome.

The key to dealing with lead poisoning is prevention. The first measure is to eliminate lead as far as possible by the substitution of alternative materials and processes. The handling of poisonous materials should be replaced by mechanical methods. A continuous campaign must be conducted against lead dusts by cleanliness, by local exhaust ventilation and by the damping of contact surfaces. Overalls must be worn at all times when at work and respirators when necessary. The workmen must be given adequate facilities for washing their hands and faces: no meals should be taken in workrooms. There should be periodic medical inspections of workpeople. Women and young persons should be excluded from the more hazardous processes.

Mercury is a liquid metal which volatizes at a moderate temperature so that the first care is to recognize and keep down the temperature of processes and even of rooms. Fumes are also produced during the heating of ores so that the preparation of mercury itself is not without hazard. Contact with the metal can cause poisoning. The making of scientific instruments, of electrical apparatus and of thermometers and barometers carries an occupational risk. Furriers and hatters use mercury compounds. There are inherent mercury risks in the chemical and pharmaceutical industries.

The signs and symptoms of chronic mercury poisoning are anaemia, salivation, gingivitis, a blue line on the gums and the loss of teeth. The organic compounds of mercury can cause dermatitis. As with lead poisoning there is a risk of pregnant women miscarrying.

Arsenic as a dust or in fumes causes irritation of the skin and mucous membranes. Gastro-intestinal irritation is followed by vomiting and a watery diarrhoea. There may be peripheral neuritis with wrist or foot drop. Coryza, conjunctivitis and laryngitis can also occur. Sixty years ago several hundred cases occurred in the north of England and were eventually traced to the contamination of beer by arsenic.

Arsenical dust and fumes are a cause of occupational skin cancer. *Arseniuretted hydrogen gas* may be accidentally produced by the interaction of an acid and metal either of which contains arsenic. The gas is extremely toxic and causes haemolysis, nausea and vomiting, albumenuria, oedema, acute peripheral sensory changes and jaundice. There may be haematuria or suppression of urine.

Carbon bisulphide is a colourless and very poisonous liquid which vaporizes at room temperature.

The vapour, when inhaled, affects the central nervous system. Acute poisoning manifests itself as mental disturbance and possibly acute mania. In chronic poisoning there is nausea, headache and giddiness with mental disturbance in the form of hysterical attacks and defective cerebration. The motor nervous system of the face, forearms and legs may be affected causing muscle weakness.

Preventive measures include fire prevention, attention to fire escape and prevention, adequate ventilation, the limitation of time of exposure and periodical medical examination.

Anilism is a syndrome of anaemia, dyspnoea, and cyanosis due to nitro and amino derivatives of benzene and toluene as well as aniline.

The characteristic blue-grey colour of the complexion due to the formation of methaemoglobin occurs before the patient feels ill. Shortness of breath is linked with the degree of anaemia followed by the sequence of delirium, convulsion and death.

The liquid derivatives of aniline, benzene and toluene are *absorbed* through the skin with great rapidity, so much so that if splashed or soaked the *immediate* first-aid measure is to remove the clothing and wash the affected skin with a suitable solvent such as acetone. Speed is essential as there is considerable risk of toxic jaundice with acute yellow atrophy of the liver.

Chronic aniline poisoning causes bladder tumours, some of which are malignant.

Aniline is associated with compounds such as dinitro-benzene, dinitrotoluene, trinitrotoluene and others used in the dyestuffs industry and the manufacture of explosives. On occasions shoe polishes containing aniline have been involved.

Great attention must be given to prevention. The first essential is to *eliminate contact* by protective close-fitting clothing, head-covering and gloves. The processes must be enclosed and mechanical procedures substituted for manual methods. Local exhaust ventilation is necessary to remove vapour or dust. There should be no dry sweeping. Young people and the unhealthy, especially alcoholics, should be excluded from this work. There should be periodic medical examinations: the workpeople employed should have a rotation of jobs so that exposure is minimized. General cleanliness is essential: washing and bathing facilities must be adequate: appropriate arrangements should be made for the rapid stripping and cleansing of those who are splashed or wetted by chemicals. It is advisable to give extra supplies of milk as a protective.

Chronic Benzene Poisoning

Benzene, a coal tar derivative, is extracted from coke-oven gas. It is used as an industrial solvent and in the chemical and explosive industries. It is also used as a motor fuel.

The major problem is the use of solvents containing benzene. There are a variety of other coal-tar distillates such as white spirit, petrol and naphtha but in practice it is the industrial use of mixtures containing benzene which constitute a serious and sometimes fatal hazard. The risk comes from exposure to the vapour in workrooms where solvents, cellulose lacquer spraying or rubber cement are used. The risk is related to the concentration and length of exposure to benzene.

Acute risks exist from the narcotic effect of inhalation in sufficient concentration of the vapour of any of the coal tar derivatives. Continual exposure to their fumes results in deterioration of general health with malaise, headache, nausea, giddiness, mild digestive disturbances and alteration in sleeping.

Benzene differs from the other distillates as it will destroy the bone marrow and so cause anaemia. The anaemia is progressive with purpura and haemorrhages from mucous membranes. The period of significant exposure can vary from a week to even years. The vapour concentration which causes poisoning is not definitely known but it is said to be anything from 200 to 5,000 parts per million. The result of the attack on the bone-marrow is a leucopenia with relative lymphocytosis.

The most effective preventive measure is to substitute other solvents for benzene and so eliminate the risk. Effective ventilation is essential. The prevention of the escape of fumes into workrooms must be vigilantly pursued.

Periodic personal blood examinations are in themselves important but take second place to the elimination or minimizing of the presence of benzene in any form.

Toxic Jaundice

This symptomatic description includes a number of syndromes due to chemical poisoning all of which have jaundice as a sequel.

Tetrachlorethane, like trinitrotoluol, causes liver damage leading to acute yellow atrophy. Low concentrations can effect a considerable proportion of those exposed. For this reason tetrachlorethane is one of the most dangerous solvents.

Carbon tetrachloride is toxic to the liver and kidneys. When used as a therapeutic agent it can have toxic effects, notably albuminuria, but recovery can take place if exposure is not prolonged.

The same effects can be caused by inhaling the vapour. When carbon tetrachloride is exposed to a flame it breaks down to form phosgene. This phenomenon becomes a risk when this form of fire extinguisher is used in a closed space. The same effect can be caused by drawing the fumes through a lighted cigarette.

Trichlorethylene like tetrachlorethane, breaks down to form phosgene when exposed to a flame. It is used as a solvent and as a dry-cleaning fluid. The main risk from trichlorethylene is its narcotic effect which comes on rapidly and which is used pharmacologically for purposes of analgesia. In consequence there is always a hazard to those working in tanks and other enclosed spaces where they can be overcome by the fumes. The analgesic effect is well known to the staff of dry-cleaning works who inhale the vapour to relieve minor painful complaints such as toothache or a 'hangover'. Trichlorethylene has no cumulative action or chronic effects.

Epitheliomatous ulceration of the skin is associated with the process in which paraffin oil, mineral oil, bitumen, pitch or tar is used. Road or roof work involving bitumen or tar, oil refinery workers and those whose clothing is apt to be soaked with lubricating oil, fuel oil or paraffin are all liable to be affected. The skin shows evidence of discoloration, dermatitis and benign or premalignant eruptions before progressing to frank epitheliomata.

Mulespinner's cancer in cotton mills is a carcinoma of scrotum or vulva resulting from long exposure to contact with lubricating oil.

Prevention is by avoiding contact with harmful substances, the use of efficient protective clothing, oil-proof barrier creams and periodic medical examination to identify pre-malignant conditions.

Chrome ulceration is associated with chromium plating, the use of bichromates and anodic oxidation. When vapour from wet processing carrying traces of chromium is inhaled the nose and especially the nasal septum are affected. When cracks in the skin are contaminated chronic ulcers called *chrome holes* are caused: they do not heal until all traces of chrome are eliminated. As the nose is not disfigured by septal ulceration it may go unrecognized until sighted on medical examination. Regulations require the provision of local exhaust ventilation over the chrome vats and the provision of rubber gloves, aprons and footwear. Adequate washing facilities are necessary. Waterproof plaster must be provided for the protection of skin cuts and abrasions. A protective ointment of vaseline and lanoline is issued for use on hands and nose. Workpeople are examined by the doctor once a fortnight and their hands and forearms twice weekly by a responsible person.

No person under eighteen may be employed in an actual chromium process or those processes following it.

Chlorinated cutting oils cause an acneform skin eruption with papules, comedones and postules. It occurs among lathe and other metal machinists and is found on the outer side of the arms, particularly around the elbow. There may be itching. The hands may also be affected causing paronychia. Prevention lies in the avoidance of the hazard by the daily issue of clean clothes and by the use of impervious protective sleeves and aprons. An oil-resistant barrier cream should also be used.

A similar condition results from work with chlorinated naphthalenes which are waxes used for electrical insulating purposes. With these there is an additional risk of toxic jaundice from the inhalation of their fumes.

Metal fume fever

When zinc is heated zinc oxide volatilizes to a fine floating dust. Inhalation produces the characteristic rigor, headache, pyrexia and sweating, not unlike the onset of malaria. There is a latent period of a few hours before the condition manifests itself. The symptoms pass off in a short time. Some acclimatization is possible.

Metal fume fever is associated with any process involving the heating of zinc. Of these the commonest is the manufacture of brass.

Manganese

Chronic manganese poisoning resembles chronic post-encephalitic parkinsonism. Those affected show emotional disturbances, monotonous voice, spastic gait and a mask-like face. The general health is not affected but the stricken are crippled for life.

The condition occurs in any process in which exposure to manganese dust is possible.

Cadmium

Cadmium, both as metal and as a salt, causes symptoms of gastro-enteritis with collapse. Poisoning has occurred after consuming citrus drinks prepared in cadmium plated vessels. Metal fumes generated in melting cadmium or cadmium alloy or in welding has a similar effect complicated by dyspnoea and an influenza-like illness. The condition can be serious or even fatal.

Industrial Dermatitis

Industrial dermatitis occurs in two categories, namely that group of conditions which are due to specific agents and the vast number of others in which no special agent is involved but which careless talk by the doctor during the initial consultation plants the idea in the patient's mind. It is a remarkable phenomenon that the vast majority of doctors, while confessing to know little of morbid conditions of the skin and having no opportunity of knowing the details of industry and its processes, on being confronted with a skin condition will frequently suggest industrial dermatitis as a differential diagnosis and thereby start that wretched, chronic and intractable psychological condition commonly known as compensation neurosis.

When eczema, scabies, syphilis and lack of soap and water have been excluded after a full examination of the whole of the patient's body it can then be borne in mind that specific dermatitis can occur in connexion with some industrial processes. It will also be recognized that there is in some degree an interaction between the specific agent, the environment and the individual. Whatever may be the circumstances of the case the preventive aspect must at once be given priority of attention, both as a means of avoiding hazard to others at risk and also as a diagnostic check, for if the measures for prevention are found to be both adequate and properly applied then the diagnosis of industrial dermatitis is doubtful: if the preventive measures are adequately planned but are not applied then the firm and its staff will be at future risk both in terms of health and in law. The doctor dealing with the case will be well advised in his own interests both to ascertain the full details of the situation and to make careful notes of them.

There are few substances in industry which, if constantly used, will not lead to dermatitis in some people. Not many people should be affected if there is a proper standard of personal cleanliness and of care of the skin.

The first preventive measure is the provision and use of adequate washing facilities. Success in their use requires the co-operation of the individual worker: this depends upon proper training and health education. Periodic medical inspection of all workpeople at risk should be carried out, more especially as it is likely that initial injury to the skin is an important causative factor.

Specific dermatitis may be due among other things to oil, petrol,

paraffin, synthetic resins and lacquers, turpentine and its sub-
stitutes, chrome, sugar, alkalis, fish, plants, flour and various
chemicals. Mites in grain, cheese, copra and other substances can
also cause skin irritation.

When the patient is removed from the process the condition
normally rapidly subsides. After appropriate treatment and the
provision of proper protection work with the original process can
often be resumed.

As many dermatological conditions are associated with removal
of the skin fat or oil such 'defatting' should be combated by the
daily use of an emollient ointment containing lanolin as an application when cleaning up after work.

Miners who often work in confined and cramped conditions
are subject to a variety of local inflammatory conditions leading to
cellulitis known as 'beat hand', 'beat elbow' or 'beat knee' according to location. These persistent conditions are associated with an
underlying bursitis.

Dust diseases

Dust diseases vary widely in their effects

1. Non-toxic inorganic dusts affecting the lungs and leading to
   silicosis.
2. Infection-carrying dusts causing anthrax, monilia and actinomycosis.
3. Irritant or corrosive dusts such as lime, arsenic, chromic
   acid, the bi-chromates.
4. Poisonous dusts such as arsenic, lead, manganese, trinitrotoluene.
5. Carcinogenic dusts such as radioactive materials, pitch,
   soot and some ores.
6. Allergic dusts resulting in a complete range of symptoms of
   allergy.

Farmer's lung

Farmer's lung is an occupational disease due to inhaling dust
carrying fungus of mouldy hay. The symptoms of dyspnoea are
rapidly relieved on removal from exposure but recur on return
to the dusty environment. Cotton workers suffer in the opening
of bales and in the carding process. So called 'cardroom worker's
asthma' is most noticeable at the beginning of the working week,

probably following the lack of exposure at the week-end. 'Weaver's cough' is another form of dust disease.

Workers in grain, hay, straw, hemp, cotton, feathers and certain hard woods suffer from the irritant effects of inhaled dust.

Bagassosis

Bagasse is the remaining fibres of the crushed cane after the sugar had been extracted. Synthetic 'insulating board' is prepared from the bagasse. The dust from the crushed cane causes a pathological lung condition.

The preventive action is to handle bagasse only in the moist state and to introduce exhaust ventilation.

Inorganic dust

Pneumonoconiosis is the fibrosis of the lung substance following the inhalation of dust. The most important inorganic dust is silica. A large variety of industries use silica-containing materials.

1. Brick-making.
2. Stone quarrying and dressing (stonemason's phthisis).
3. Metal grinding (grinder's rot).
4. Sand blasting.
5. Pottery manufacture (potter's asthma).
6. Silica crushing and grinding.
7. Mining through rock whether for metal, ore, coal or in building tunnels.

Silicosis is due to the lodging of silica dust SiO_2 in the lung alveoli with subsequent biological action leading to lung fibrosis with the occurrence of dyspnoea which becomes chronic. Diagnosis is aided by chest X-Ray. Death is usually due to broncho-pneumonia secondary to influenza. Pulmonary tuberculosis is a common complication.

Asbestosis

Asbestosis occurs following the inhalation of asbestos dust over a long period. Asbestos is a silicate and the disease resembles silicosis though there are some pathological differences. Tuberculosis is a less common complication.

Prevention of pneumonoconiosis is essentially the control of the dust hazard. Wherever possible the elimination of silica is an ideal as, for example, the substitution of *shot* blasting for *sand* blasting and the replacement of flint by alumina in the preparation of pottery. Dust should be suppressed especially by the use of water. Local exhaust ventilation should be arranged at the back of machines so that the dust is sucked away and prevented from entering the general atmosphere of the workroom. The use of respirators and positive pressure helmets is secondary to efficient extractor ventilation and not a replacement for it. The general health of the workpeople involved should be overseen by initial and periodic medical examinations.

Caisson disease

The mechanical versatility of man now requires him to work under conditions of alteration of atmospheric pressure varying from the high pressures of deep sea diving or equivalent civil engineering work in air locks under pressure to the rarefied atmospheric conditions of high altitude flying. The conditions represent the extremes of a graph of pressure with normal atmospheric pressure as a mean.

Caisson disease is the result of the sudden transition from an atmosphere of sustained high pressure to normal atmospheric pressure. Before workmen enter the chamber or caisson where work is done they pass through an air lock in which the pressure is rapidly raised to that in the interior or the caisson. When it is time to leave they re-enter the air-lock. The pressure within is then *gradually* reduced at a rate laid down in physiological tables so that the nitrogen element of high pressure air leaves the body gradually and comes out of solution in the tissues without forming minute bubbles which could damage the brain or other parts of the body. A sudden release of pressure after lengthy exposure usually causes an attack of 'bends' within minutes or hours. These are characterized by severe pain in muscles and joints. Paralysis of the legs, retention of urine, abdominal pain, vertigo and nose bleeding are noted. In severe cases bubbles forming in the brain and spinal cord produce a variety of neurological phenomena.

Prevention is by selection, education and training and careful attention to the procedures for compression and decompression. Healthy men aged 20 to 30 with no heart or lung trouble and free of catarrh should be selected: alcoholics should be excluded.

The length of working shifts and decompression routines of the latest Royal Navy diving tables should be adhered to. The air supplied to the caisson should be pure and cooled if necessary.

Treatment of 'bends' is by recompression and slow decompression in a warmed air lock under medical supervision.

In addition to caisson disease other complications occur when working under high pressure. Catarrh or other blockage of the Eustachian tube causes extreme pain and possible damage when the pressure is raised at the outset. The sinuses may be affected at the same time. If the subject persists in being exposed to increasing pressure septic material may enter the middle ear from the Eustachian tube with resultant infection.

Similar conditions occur with deep sea diving. As the diving dress acts as a pneumatic cushion to protect the diver from the pressure of the water there is a special risk when divers fall from a height while under water, as for example, off a sunken wreck. The sudden and immense increase of pressure due to the increased depth cannot be immediately compensated so there is a 'squeeze' which is a painful condition of the chest and upper limbs with minor nervous changes.

Compressed air tools have an open exhaust. The escaping air can enter the tissues and split them if there is access through a skin wound. This is relatively harmless compared with the consequences of trauma caused in the hand and forearm by the entry under pressure of grease from lubrication grease guns. A new industrial device is the explosive powered 'gun' which fires bolts into concrete or through steel plate. This weapon is as risky as any other firearm used in a confined space.

Electrocution

Electrocution is an occupational hazard extending far beyond the bounds of the electrical industry. Even setting aside domestic accidents the risk exists wherever electricity is present or is in use. Broken wires, poor insulation, faulty connexions and the like are obvious risks but others exist by the interposition of an unexpected conductor such as a metal ladder brought into contact with some live bare metal conductor.

The danger in electricity is in its power. The *voltage* is of little consequence: it is the *amperage* which is significant. Extremely high voltage electricity flows over the surface of conductors: when the body is made to be a conductor the same phenomenon occurs. Alternating current is more dangerous than direct current in that the body is subject to a repeating bombardment of reversing electric currents by the alternating system: direct current exposes the body to only one stimulus. If the current is sufficient either variety will kill. The effects of electrocution are damage to the central nervous system and local burning. The immediate result is to render the patient unconscious. First aid consists of stopping further exposure by interrupting the current and then applying artifical respiration to restore breathing.

Accident prevention in industry

While much can be written about specific clinical conditions due to occupation yet the vast majority of occupational ill health is due to an immense variety of non-specific happenings causing some form of trauma. These can be visualized rather than described. The workman on an unswept floor stumbles over a minor obstruction, treads on a nail concealed by paper or kneels on some sharp object which penetrates the knee joint. Walking under a hazard something falls on him. An unguarded opening engulfs him. A loose hammer head flies off and hits him. Heads of tools such as chisels develop feather-like splinters which can penetrate the hand or, if broken off, will enter an eye. Poor lifting techniques mean strained backs. Ladders with defective or missing rungs cause falls. Defective slings allow objects to fall. Men working on roofs are luckier if they fall through asbestos rather than glass. Tools and heavy objects drop on to the unprotected feet and crush them. Unguarded machines mangle hands. Workpeople are drawn into machinery if their clothing is slack or if their hair is long. Exposure to red heat causes eye cataract. Sharp tools are always a risk. Poor lighting conceals hazards.

There is no cure for accidents: there is only prevention. This depends upon health education.

15

Radiation and Health

RADIATION became significant to health at the end of the nineteenth century with the introduction of X-Rays by Roentgen, the discovery by Becquerel of the radio-activity of uranium and the work of the Curie family on radium.

Radiation is associated with atomic structure and occurs as

X-Rays
Gamma rays
Alpha particles
Beta particles
Neutrons.

The effect of radiation is due to the ability of all the above (except the neutron) when passing through any material to knock an *electron out of its orbit* in the constituent atoms. By such impact the radiation loses energy. The dislocation of the electron is known as *ionization* as the result is to form two *ions*, the one made up of the mutilated atom minus its electron (and positively charged) and the other, the electron alone (negatively charged) which then attaches itself to a neutral atom.

The phenomenon of ionization is the method by which radiation causes physical, chemical or biological change.

The simplest way to measure any radiation would be in terms of the number of particles striking a given area in a given time. Then, if a particular square centimetre of body tissue was being struck by 100 beta particles per second, one might be led to think that twice as much damage was being done as, say, on a neighbouring part which was only getting 50 particles per second. But this way of measuring by itself is not enough. What we are interested in is the number of ions produced, and this depends on the energy of the incident particles as well as on their number.

It is useful to measure radiation in terms of the ionization it produces. The unit used is the *roentgen*. For convenience in dealing with smaller quantities of radiation the roentgen is divided into 1000 milli-roentgen (mr).

The roentgen is a measure of the number of ions produced per c.c. This means that the total damage done to a given organism by a given dose in roentgens depends on the volume over which the radiation is applied, for example, a dose of 2,000r which was confined to a subject's big toe would not do very much harm except to the big toe, but the same dose applied over the whole of his body would certainly be lethal.

The roentgen is a measure of the number of ions per c.c. in air. Body tissue is something like a thousand times as dense as air, and a roentgen will accordingly produce about a thousand times as many ions per c.c. in it. (The roentgen is defined in terms of the numbers of ions produced per c.c. in air because this can be measured without very much difficulty, whereas the number of ions produced in tissue cannot.)

The roentgen is a measure of total dose. Dose-rate can be measured in r per minute or r per hour. It should be noted that the roentgen was originally intended for measuring doses of X- or gamma radiation. It can be used to measure alpha and beta particle doses too, but a dose of 1 r of either of these, because of their short range and consequent heavy surface effect, will have a different effect in tissue from a dose of 1 r of X-rays.

The relative persistence of radiation is estimated in relation to the length of time it takes half the atoms of the radio-active material to disintegrate: this is called the *half life*. The time varies from an instant to millions of years. If at the end of one period the material loses half its activity then at the end of a second equal period the surviving half will itself have been halved to leave a quarter: at the end of the third period this quarter will itself be halved and so on.

It will be seen at once that the shorter the half life the more energetic will be the disintegration of the atoms and conversely the longer the half life the longer will be the emission of effective radiation. The biological result to the human patient is that with a too short half life a radioactive therapeutic substance breaks up prematurely while a material which has too long a half life and is retained overlong in the tissues as a source of radiation may be active long enough to become carcinogenic. To be of therapeutic value a radioactive substance should have a half life of twelve hours to fourteen days.

The *effective* amount of radiation received by the tissues depends upon the *amount* of the radio-active material and the *rate* of disintegration. This latter figure is measured in *curies* defined as the amount of radio-active material in which $3 \cdot 7 \times 10^{10}$ disintegrations occur in one second. It is based on the rate of disintegration of one gram of radium. As this is too big a unit for general use, a *millicurie* is defined as the thousandth part of a curie ($3 \cdot 7 \times 10^7$) and a *microcurie* ($3 \cdot 7 \times 10^4$) as the millionth part of a curie.

Personal measurement of radiation is made by:

(a) A *personal dosimeter* which is a tubular instrument like a fountain pen. It is essentially an electroscope graduated to indicate the ionization which causes it to discharge. It can be calibrated and it shows at once if the wearer is risking an overdose.

(b) *Film badges.* These miniature photographic films are blackened by the effects of radiation, the amount of blackening shown after developing being proportionate to the exposure.

(c) *Particle counters.* Used for the detection of low-activity gamma-ray emitters.
     (i) Geiger counter.
     (ii) Scintillation counter.

Radiation is used for many peaceful purposes in medicine, in industry and for scientific investigations.

In medicine X-Rays are used for diagnosis and treatment. Radium is a therapeutic agent. Radio-isotopes are used for external radiotherapy. Isotopes are also given by mouth or injection to direct the radio-active material to accumulate in some tissue requiring limited local attack: a typical example is the administration of radio-active iodine with the intention of concentrating radio-activity in the tissues of the thyroid gland. In the same way a pathological bone marrow or a carcinoma metastasis may be selectively attacked. Isotopes can also be used for diagnosis by tracking their progress in the tissues.

Industry uses X-Rays to detect flaws in metal work. Thickness and unevenness may also be measured. Leak detection in pipe systems is now possible. Foods and pharmaceutical products can be sterilized.

In research radio-activity is used in a variety of processes from engineering to entomology in order to follow routes and spread which otherwise would be either tedious or impossible.

158 PUBLIC AND COMMUNITY HEALTH

Radiation Hazards

The side effects of X-Rays and radium were recognized soon after their introduction, the commonest being an erythema which preceded radiation burns and the early occupational mutilation of radiologists. Although radiation protective devices such as shielding were introduced, the effect was found to be cumulative and the significant factor the *maximum permissible* dose (MPD).

Radiation Protection

There are two basic protection factors, namely the *length of time* of exposure and the *distance* from the source which is significant as the intensity is reduced in proportion to the square of the distance.

Shielding of the source can be provided. If manipulation of the material is required this can be carried out from a distance under indirect control and observation. It is essential that personnel should be aware of the principles of radio-activity and of safe handling of sources so that they can anticipate risks and apply safety measures in an intelligent manner. The precautions against contamination must be clearly understood by all and rehearsed as necessary.

External radiation from the source must be controlled. Sources are either sealed or unsealed, the latter producing more complicated safety problems. Contamination from an unsealed source of radio-active material is in the form of splashes, drips or leaks or the escape of vapour or dust. This requires the provision of double containers to take up escaping material and arrangements for processing or storage in fume cupboards. Protective gloves and gowns should be worn as well as eyeshields where necessary. Firm industrial discipline must be applied to the work routines, including the proper segregation, use and disposal of equipment, materials and waste and such conduct as the total prohibition of smoking, drinking and eating in the workplace.

Waste disposal methods have to be considered in relation to the public health when it is proposed to discharge vapour to the air or when dealing with liquid or solid sources.

The Clinical Effects of Radiation Hazards

Background radiation from natural sources must not be forgotten in assessing overall clinical effects.

External sources are:
Cosmic rays
Natural radiation substances in the environment.

Internal sources include:
Body constituents.
Potassium 40
Carbon 14
Radium
Thorium

Man-made radiation
Diagnostic and therapeutic radiology.
Radio-active isotopes used in research and industry.
Luminous dial painting.
Industrial radiography.
X-Ray shoe fitting.
High power television sets.
Radio-active fall-out from nuclear weapon testing.
Direct effects of nuclear weapons.
Radio-active waste from the use and processing of radio-active
materials and fission products.
Accidental release of radio-active substances.

Effects of radiation on the tissues
Somatic: Genetic.
The effects of ionizing radiation.
Alpha and *low energy beta* radiations do not penetrate the skin
and so are not a hazard from the exterior.
High energy beta radiation (e.g. Strontium 90) can penetrate the
skin and reach the germinal layer.
Bone is affected by penetrating radiation which can overcome
the resistant barrier of the calcium in the bone and attack the
sensitive marrow. The bone itself can undergo necrosis and
spontaneous fracture.
The testes and ovaries are very sensitive to radiation, which
causes reduced sperm production, amenorrhoea and sterility, the
latter usually temporary unless massive doses of radiation are
received.
The gastro-intestinal tract epithelium is affected by radiation
leading to degeneration and loss of specific function followed by

ulceration. The loss of the protective mucosa invites infection and haemorrhage. Irritation of the mucosa promotes a response by diarrhoea and fluid loss.

The blood forming organs, bone marrow, lymphatic system and in the foetus the spleen and in children the thymus react to acute or chronic radiation attack.

1. Acute
   Depression of formation of white cells and platelets.
   Red cells live longer: any destructive process is delayed.
2. Chronic (usually by bone-seeking radio-isotopes).
   Aplastic anaemia.
   Aleukaemic leukaemia.

Observation is by routine differential blood count to see the effect on the white cells. It should be noted that an initial blood count should always be made before starting on a job involving radiation: this is to exclude other pathological conditions which existed before radiation exposure but which would be attributed to radiation if no evidence existed before exposure.

The eyes, if subject to excessive radiation, may develop cataract. This phenomenon may be a complication of radio-therapy.

The lungs are liable to develop fibrosis when exposed to heavy radiation doses as for example when radio-therapy is given to check or destroy a carcinoma of the lung. A similar condition is recognized in uranium miners exposed to radon gas.

The central nervous system is relatively insensitive to the effects of radiation.

The foetus is significantly sensitive to radiation which can unbalance its development leading to abnormality or even its loss by abortion. Radiation attacks the stage of growth which is active at the time of exposure. As the most significant foetal development takes place in the first two months of pregnancy it is at this period that radiation bombardment can result in the grossest abnormalities. In the later months of pregnancy quite small doses of radiation can affect the still incomplete foetal central nervous system.

Clinical radiographic examinations of the pregnant woman, particularly of her pelvis, can expose the foetus in utero to damaging doses of radiation. It is quite possible that radio-active material ingested by the mother if suitable for absorption by special tissues in the foetus such as the thyroid will accumulate there as a focus of radio-activity and consequent later damage.

Irradiation of the Whole Body/Acute Effects

The *mean lethal dose* MDL for a single acute episode of exposure of the whole body is 200–900 r. This is the dose which would kill half of those exposed to it. Massive doses considerably greater than this will cause *biological collapse* with gross tissue destruction, shock, coma and death in a few hours.

The progression of the acute radiation syndrome to ultimate death is seen with doses of 500–1000 r. In such cases death is due to intestinal or haemopoietic damage.

There are four stages:

(a) A brief symptomless latent period.

(b) Nausea and vomiting occurring within a few hours and passing off in 24 hours, succeeded by malaise, lassitude, diarrhoea and thirst, anorexia and drowsiness for about a week

(c) A secondary period of apparent well-being except for malaise, anorexia and a minor pyrexia.

(d) At the end of the third week there is sudden epilation: in the fourth week gross and possibly terminal symptoms appear. There is increasing malaise and fever with the occurrence of agranulocytic angina and necrotic gingivitis with pain, oedema, inflammation, ulceration and bleeding from gums. There is an onset of general haemorrhage with purpura, epistaxis, a bloody diarrhoea and, in women, metrorrhagia. There is leucopenia and a reduced platelet count. If the patient survives this stage he may recover or die from delayed gastro-intestinal conditions or from a chronic sepsis which the body, now unable to produce leucocytes, cannot resist. The patient may sink and die in a condition of exhaustion, diarrhoea and emaciation.

Treatment of Acute Radiation of the Whole Body

At the present time treatment is supportive and symptomatic. Blood transfusion preferably with fresh blood enriched with platelets will offer a temporary period of blood adequacy until the haemopoietic system has a chance to recover and to start repopulation with new blood cells. Normal marrow has been given from donors with promising initial results.

M

Radiation-induced Cancer

Cancer was early recognized as a hazard among the first generation of radiologists. The original risk from unprotected sources was radiation-induced dermatitis followed in a few years by skin cancer.

Carcinoma of the lung has always been an occupational disease among uranium miners of the Schneeburg and Joachimstal. In New York there was a classic epidemic of bone sarcoma in painters using luminous paint for watch dials and shaping the tips of brushes on their lips.

Post-cricoid carcinoma has occurred after X-Ray therapy of carcinoma of the thyroid. Similarly in children cancer of the thyroid has followed the administration of small doses of radiation to the gland. The fashionable therapeutic use of radio-active spa water a generation ago has left carcinoma of the stomach as a sequel.

Radiation and Leukaemia

Leukaemia has resulted from exposure to radiation
(a) In radiologists working unshielded.
(b) Following heavy therapeutic doses of radiation, e.g. ankylosing spondylitis.
(c) In those exposed to atomic bomb attack in Japan.
(d) In children who were exposed to repeated diagnostic radiation *in utero*.

Genetic effects of radiation

The genetic effects of radiation cannot be accurately assessed though they are of the greatest significance. Radiation which attacks chromosomes can interfere with the process of mutation so that one or more genes are displaced.

Radiation hazards inside the body

Radio-active substances can enter the body by
Ingestion.
Inhalation.
Break in skin continuity.
Injection.

The effect of the substance depends upon the quantity and also the biological half-life. Depending upon the body chemistry these radio-active substances tend to have affinities for certain specific tissues. The effect of such a radio-active substance must be estimated in relation to the result of its action on a special part of the body such as the thyroid gland.

The commoner isotopes which affect the body tissue are as follows:

Bone Marrow
Phosphorus 32
Tritium 3H
Sodium 24
Chlorine 36
Thyroid
Iodine 131
Bone
Radium 226
Plutonium ... ... 239 (Soluble)
Strontium 90
Calcium 45
Lungs
Radon gas 222
Plutonium ... ... 239 (Insoluble)
Kidneys
Gold 138
Uranium and other heavy metals.

The *maximum permissible dose of radiation* is the greatest which does not cause appreciable injury.

The maximum permissible dose of X-Rays or Gamma rays to the whole body over a period of 10 years should not exceed 50 r. nor should more than 5 r. be received in any period of 12 months.

Those occupationally exposed to radiation should not receive more than 100 mr a week.

The permissible weekly dose to others is 100 mr to bone, bone marrow, eyes, gonads 600 mr to skin

Detection of radio-active isotopes in the body
Gamma radiation by Geiger counter
Beta radiation of excretion studies of breath, urine.

Treatment of Accidental Contamination
Eyes, hands Wash: test with Geiger counter
Ingestion Stomach washout: purge
Try to render insoluble in gut.

Chelating agents such as *ethylene diamine tetra acetic acid* (EDTA) may help in removing radio-active substances from the body.

The Hazard from low-level radiation

Background radiation has been estimated at

Bone ...   .   125 mr/year
Gonads, bone marrow, soft tissue 95 mr/year

Radiation in water from radium or mesothorium is cumulative in bone: radiation in food consists of alpha-particle activity, most of which is excreted in forty-eight hours. These levels are of negligible significance except to the armchair expert otherwise the whole process of eating food would be highly dangerous.

Man-made radiation

Annual doses

Natural background	85–106 mr
Diagnostic radiology (UK 1957)	19 mr
Occupational exposure	0·5 mr
Fall-out (1958–59)	2·4 mr
Miscellaneous	less than one

It is only the long half-life isotopes of fall-out which are of significance (Caesium 137 Strontium 90 Carbon 14).

Danger to Individuals

Man-made additional risks are negligible. Even to those occupationally involved the personal risk, except for accidents, is very small due to adequate preventive, protective and training measures.

Genetic effects on the total population

The significant radiation dose is the *average* one to the entire potential child-bearing population. Any addition to radiation is significant in proportion to its size and will add to the genetic burden.

Danger from radio-active fall-out

The chief danger is Strontium 90 as a cause of bone sarcoma. The risk is negligibly low compared with the other hazards of life, when the episode is limited to occasional weapon testing or accident at an atomic station.

Danger from diagnostic radiology

This danger is associated with the degree of skill, insight and forethought of the radiologist and technicians. Dosage is proportionate to the *time of exposure*. Good first exposures avoid retakes each with its cumulative increase in X-Ray exposure.

Mass miniature radiography, due to the intensity and scatter of its rays, may lead to undesirable exposure or dosing of children and pregnant women. In consequence, these latter groups should not normally be examined by mass X-Ray. If examination is essential then it should be by a full-size plate which gives a lesser dose of radiation.

Diagnostic radiography of the chest is a valuable preventive measure in keeping control of and excluding those with demonstrable chest tuberculosis from infecting children and others at special risk.

Annual chest X-Ray presents negligible risk to the individual: in any case the procedure is planned to protect others, especially children, from a much greater hazard of tuberculosis.

Atomic warfare and public health

A war cannot be fought without incurring casualties or damage. The decisions of war are not medical but are political or philosophical. It must be remembered that Europe survived the Black Death without any medico-social services or tangible links with the rest of the world. The atomic threat is not one of population elimination but of massive attacks on large targets which do not represent the whole or even the major part of the population of the country. The essential task is to preserve the next generation and to restore a normal way of life in the country. Humanitarian effort in dealing with casualties is secondary to this fundamental issue.

Atomic warfare means the infliction on the civil population of the equivalent of a series of artificial earthquakes complicated by the subsequent 'fall-out' of radio-active dust, rain or other precipitation. The public health problems arise from

(a) Pre-war evacuation of priority classes of civilians.
(b) Bombing with consequent mass casualties.
(c) The public health problems of radio-active fall-out.
(d) The rescue of casualties and caring for the homeless.
(e) The restoration of a normal way of life.

Health problems include:

(a) Adequacy and safety of water and food supplies.
(b) Hygiene and sanitation.
(c) Casualties, including the disposal of the dead.
(d) Incidental illness.

This task is complicated by

(a) Shortages of trained personnel.
(b) Lack of transport.
(c) Demand upon public utility services.
(d) Inadequate hospital services.
(e) Restriction on movement.
(f) Lowered public morale.
(g) Breakdown of public control.

Pre-war evacuation of selected civilians

Selection for evacuation and despatch would be according to a prepared plan of priorities and should aim at the preservation intact of all future citizens. This means the evacuation of schoolchildren, adolescents, mothers with pre-school children, and expectant mothers. In addition all hospital patients unable to return home would be evacuated as well as any health and education staff who could be spared.

Reception arrangements must include emergency feeding and shelter, infectious disease control, general medical care and, after billeting is completed, the provision of information services and the restoration of education facilities, possibly on a shift system. A further problem is the provision of occupation of large groups of adolescents who would otherwise find themselves without work or means.

The consequences of bombing

The explosion of an atomic bomb causes an immediate liberation of radio-activity in the so-called 'gamma-flash' together with blast and fire from the intense heat generated. The liberated radio-activity is absorbed within a given radius or is dispersed in the dust and debris thrown into the upper atmosphere to be carried by the prevailing winds and then, after due delay, to fall back to earth where its radio-activity constitutes a new danger. The blast causes every type of injury as well as widespread destruction to buildings.

The heat causes flash burns of exposed body surfaces and secondary burns of any degree or extent. It ignites anything in range that will burn and heats up those materials which will not burn. The radiation causes early radiation sickness as well as delayed effects and long-term injuries.

Modern military thought implies the use of megaton bombs. The explosive effects of these is so devastating that the range of effect of the 'gamma-flash' is exceeded by that of massive and fatal damage by blast or fire. The radiation hazard is therefore limited to those within the effective radius of explosion who have survived blast and fire by taking refuge in shelters, deep cellars or tunnels. The picture is one of mass conventional casualties due to blast or fire on the periphery of the explosion and of surviving groups awaiting rescue or evacuation from safe cover in the central irradiated area where they are inaccessible to rescuers until the overlying barrier of radiation has decreased in intensity.

The organization for casualties is based upon a preliminary sorting by mobile Forward Medical Aid Units and the passing back to appropriate services. The hospitals in intact areas would be reinforced by Army medical units and expanded by the taking over of any suitable accommodation. Ambulant cases would be given domiciliary care. The initial help comes from the local authority Ambulance Service expanded into the First Aid and Ambulance Section of Civil Defence and organized as mobile columns to be deployed at a distance.

The disposal of casualties depends on the overall situation, bearing in mind the danger from radio-active fall-out and the need to avoid unnecessary over-exposure of civil defence personnel to radiation which is cumulative in its effects. The whole strength of the Civil Defence Service cannot be deployed to the full in the first episode otherwise no strategic reserve is available for later happenings.

Public Health Problems of Fall-Out

Radiological fall-out is distributed to leeward of the explosion as a plume of contamination over a leaf-shaped area in much the same way as the visible smoke is carried from a chimney by a strong wind. The precipitation comes down after an interval depending upon the wind speed and the distance down wind of the explosion. The amount of radio-activity in fall-out can be observed and its decay calculated.

Individual protection depends upon taking cover in premises which shield the occupants from radiation. Shielding is by the interposition of a resistant material such as concrete, lead, brickwork or a thick layer of earth. Alternatively, as the intensity of the radiation decreases according to the inverse square law, it is sufficient if the radio-activity is held off by the thin roof and walls of a conventional house provided that the inhabitants take refuge in a cellar or fall-out shelter. In these circumstances the distance between the radio-activity and the refuge is itself a protection. Evacuation of those under cover is a problem for the Civil Defence Controller who estimates the intensity of local radiation and takes action to arrange evacuation as soon as this is possible.

Apart from personal risk fall-out will affect water, food, animals and crops. Preservable foodstuffs can be cleared by secluded storage until its radio-activity has gone. In the same way storage reservoirs of water can be cleared by being left alone. Animals are exposed to the same risks as human beings and must be given similar protection. Standing crops may clear of radiation before they ripen but on the other hand they may suffer growth damage.

The most pressing task after checking the water supply is to monitor stocks of food which are in shops or stores and which are needed for immediate consumption. If actual contact has been avoided then theoretically there is no risk. It is desirable to remove surface layers of such items as cheeses or the top layer of paper-topped jars or packets of butter.

In general foodstuffs to which fall-out dust has no access are safe but the access of fall-out makes food dangerous until it has been monitored and pronounced safe. Food stored in sealed cartons, in refrigerators and sealed cold storage chambers may be regarded as safe as is tinned and bottled food. It has been suggested that to provide a temporary stock of safe drinking water during a period of fall-out brewery plants which pack beer in tins should divert their canning plant to packing water on the real imminence of war.

The safety of food and drink in atomic war must be settled locally and will be the responsibility of the health department.

Rescue of casualties and caring for the homeless

The problems of rescue are largely determined by the intensity of radiation in permitting access. The homeless, whether casualties or not, will require accommodation. This immediately poses questions of hygiene in terms of the large scale establishment of latrines and the disposal of excreta, the hygiene of rest centres and of emergency feeding, food handling and storage and of refuse disposal. Refugees will have to be accommodated in intact areas. The proposed allocation of at least one family to a room will bring with it all the circumstances of the days of the Industrial Revolution to a nation accustomed to being cherished by a Welfare State.

The restoration of a normal way of life

The overpowering emotions of the moment will make the days of nuclear crisis acceptable to the population. Afterwards the citizens of a land riven by bombing, disrupted in its way of life and with many facilities destroyed will have to cope with the rebuilding of the nation without the advantages of unhindered overseas trade and food imports.

A series of medico-social priorities will have to be determined including nutrition, infant and child health rehousing and the rehabilitation of the maimed.

INDEX

170